BMA

FAMILY DOCTOR GUIDES

Gallstones and Liver Problems

Dr Malcolm Bateson

Series editor: Dr Tony Smith

Dr Bateson is a consultant physician and specialist in gastroenterology in Bishop Auckland, Co. Durham

EQUATION

Published by Equation in association with the British Medical Association

First published 1988

British Library Cataloguing in Publication Data

Bateson, Malcolm
Gallstones and liver problems.
1. Man. Biliary tract. Diseases
I. Title   II. Series
616.3'6

ISBN 1-85336-077-5

Picture acknowledgements
John Rae: pp. 15, 51, 58, 75; Westminster Hospital CT Scanning
unit: pp. 83, 84; Regional Medical Physics Dept., Dryburn
Hospital, Durham: pp. 27, 42, 93; David Woodroffe: diagrams;
Derek Marriott: cartoons.

Titles in the series:

Confusion in Old Age
Gallstones and Liver Problems
Arthritis
Asthma
Children's Health 1–5
Strokes and their Prevention

Typeset by Columns of Reading
Printed and bound in Great Britain
by The Bath Press, Avon.

Equation , Wellingborough, Northamptonshire NN8 2RQ, England.

10 9 8 7 6 5 4 3 2 1

Contents

1 INTRODUCTION   7
Some anatomical features of the liver; What
the gallbladder does; What the liver does;
What can make the liver go wrong?; What the
pancreas does; What the spleen does

2 WHAT CAN GO WRONG WITH THE LIVER?   19
Jaundice; Fluid; Bleeding;
Itch and diarrhoea; Mental problems

3 WHAT CAN GO WRONG WITH THE PANCREAS?   25
Inflammation of the pancreas; Acute pancreatitis;
Chronic pancreatitis; Cancer

4 WHAT CAN GO WRONG WITH THE
GALLBLADDER AND BILE DUCTS?   27
Gallstone disease; How bile is made;
The gallbladder at work; What's in the bile?

5 HOW GALLSTONES FORM   31
A delicate balance; It takes more than
cholesterol; Crystals; Bilirubin

6 WHO GETS GALLSTONES?   34
Race and country; Age; Female sex;
Overweight; Diet; Drugs; Anaemia; Gallstones
are common

7 HOW DO GALLSTONES SHOW UP?   40
Sometimes there are no symptoms;
When there are symptoms

8 HOW DO YOU FIND GALLSTONES?   42
Ultrasound; Oral cholecystogram; Other tests;
Blood tests; Does the gallbladder get diseased
without stones?; When do gallstones matter?
Finding gallstones unexpectedly; When
gallstones cause symptoms

9 HOW DO YOU TREAT GALLSTONES?   47
Treatment for pain; Surgery for gallstones;
How the operation is done; Do people get
cured?; Fashions in treatment; Is diet treatment

useful for gallstones?; Dissolving gallstones;
Bile duct stones; Smashing ideas for the
future; Ether treatment makes a comeback;
What about gallbladder cancer?

10 ALCOHOL AND LIVER DISEASE   58

Drinking habits in different countries; Safe limits;
How alcohol affects the liver; How your liver
adapts; How your liver is damaged; How the
doctor knows you are a heavy drinker; Tests;
Can alcoholism be treated?

11 VIRUSES AND LIVER DISEASE   68

Hepatitis A; Protection from the virus; Hepatitis B;
Another infection; How does it spread?;
Hepatitis non-A non-B; Other viruses; Glandular
fever; Other problems

12 AUTO-IMMUNE LIVER DISEASE   77

Primary biliary cirrhosis; Chronic active hepatitis

13 POISONS, DRUGS AND HERBS   79

Carbon tetrachloride; Paracetamol; Anaesthesia;
Tranquillisers; Sex hormones; Herbs

14 TREATMENT OF LIVER FAILURE   82

What can be done? Transplants

15 LIVER CANCER   83

How is it treated? Secondary liver cancer

16 TESTS FOR LIVER DISEASE   85

Physical signs; Blood tests; Bilirubin; Enzymes;
Albumin; Globulin; Cholesterol; Urea; Electrolytes;
Blood count; Viral infections; Other tests;
Red herrings

17 LIVER BIOPSY   90

How it is done

18 WHY ON EARTH DID I GO YELLOW?   91

The possibilities; Tests

19 X RAYS AND SCANS   93

X rays; Isotope scan; Ultrasound

20 CONCLUSION   95

    INDEX   96

1 Introduction

Few people without medical training have much idea what the liver does. It is fairly easy to understand the functions of the heart (a blood pump), the kidneys (which get rid of waste by forming urine), and the stomach (digestion of food), but the liver's job cannot be explained in a few words.

Yet the liver is the biggest single organ in the body — and is essential to life. Its prime job is to act as the storehouse and processing plant for the nutrients extracted from food and drink by the intestines. All the blood that leaves the stomach and intestines (loaded with sugars, peptides, and other food products) goes into the liver before returning to the heart, and it is in the liver that our bodies make first use of the food we eat.

The liver also plays a part in the digestive process; some of its own factory wastes are converted into a mixture, bile, which helps in the breakdown of fatty foods. Bile is stored until needed in the gallbladder.

The bile duct — the narrow tube through which bile is emptied from the gallbladder — enters the intestine at the same point as another duct or tube leading from the pancreas. The pancreas produces many of the digestive juices (as well as the hormone insulin).

The liver, gallbladder, and pancreas are so close together that disease in one may affect the others, so this book looks at all three — in health and disease.

Some anatomical features of the liver

The liver is triangular in shape and weighs about 1½kg (over 3 lb). It sits just beneath the diaphragm, the curved flat muscle below the lungs, which is used in breathing. Most of the liver is on your right side and your doctor can feel it under your ribs while you are breathing in. Because the liver is much larger than is absolutely necessary, parts can be removed without harming your health. The liver tends to be smaller in women and it also gets smaller with age, but this does not mean that it works less well.

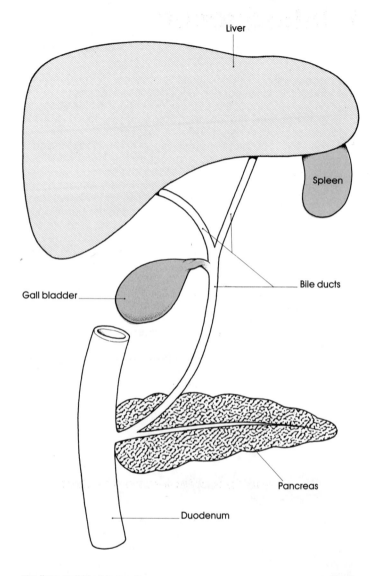

The liver, gall bladder and pancreas.

Two blood supplies

Oxygen, energy, and substances for processing are carried to the liver in the blood and waste products are removed in the same way. The liver gets its blood from two different places — from the heart (via the hepatic artery) and the intestines (via the portal vein). The hepatic artery supplies the oxygen-rich blood, while the portal vein brings blood from the intestines containing breakdown products of food.

Within the liver the blood flows along spaces called sinusoids and is collected in tiny veins which join to form the hepatic vein, which takes the blood back to the heart.

The liver showing blood supply.

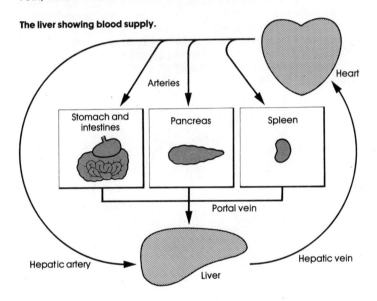

Two outlets

The liver has two outlets. Firstly, it can send chemicals and other substances through the hepatic vein and so into the bloodstream. But each liver cell also makes the fluid called bile. Bile is collected through a system of tiny tubes which join to form larger tubes and eventually form the right and left hepatic bile ducts. These two ducts join in turn to make the common hepatic duct, which then becomes the common bile duct when it joins the cystic duct from the gallbladder, and takes bile to the beginning of the small intestine, which is called the duodenum.

What the gallbladder does

A side tube opens off the common (main) bile duct. This branch, the cystic duct, leads to the gallbladder, a bag the size of a large plum that can store bile until it is needed, when its muscular wall will squeeze the bile out quickly. The gallbladder lies on the right-hand side of the abdomen, under the liver, tucked out of harm's way.

The common bile duct enters the duodenum (small intestine) next to the duct which drains the pancreas, so that the two ducts share the opening into the intestines. The pancreas lies at the back of the abdomen, across the spine. At the point in the duodenal wall where these ducts enter there is a muscle ring called the papilla or ampulla; this can act as a valve to control the flow of bile and prevent fluid from the duodenum flowing back into the bile duct and the pancreatic duct.

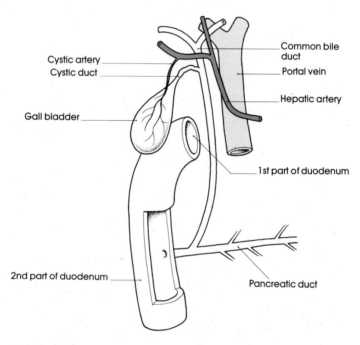

The biliary system.

Bile

Bile is a mixture of acids, pigments, and the fatty substance called cholesterol. When bile enters the intestine some of these chemicals are passed out of the body in the stools. The bile acids — which help to absorb fats — are largely reabsorbed into the blood, however, and so are passed back to the liver through the portal vein. The liver can then use them again when it forms fresh bile. This process goes under the grand name of the enterohepatic circulation, which only means that the bile acids go round and round inside you.

What the liver does

As I said at the beginning of the book, the liver performs a host of essential jobs, which is why it is so important to look after it well.

It's a factory

The liver makes:
- **Albumin (a protein)**
- **Clotting factors**
- **Bile acids, which help to absorb fats and vitamins A, D, and K**

The liver is a factory that makes substances the body needs, such as the protein called albumin, which helps the circulation work properly and carries other things around the bloodstream. The liver makes a whole number of protein clotting factors which help your blood to stop flowing when you cut yourself.

The bile acids are produced from cholesterol in the liver. They pass into the intestine through the bile ducts and gallbladder and help to absorb fats and the vitamins that can dissolve in fats — vitamins A (for night vision), D (which builds strong bones), and K (which helps blood clot properly).

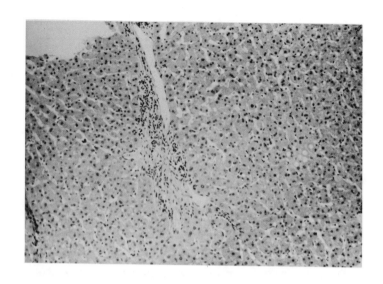

The normal liver, above, has its cells arranged in a regular pattern. In the diseased liver, below, much of the organ has been replaced by fat and scar tissue.

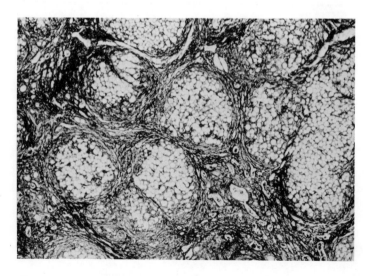

It's a regulator

The liver regulates the amount of cholesterol in the bloodstream. Cholesterol is a fat-like substance which is an essential part of all animal cells, and is also needed to make hormones (chemical messengers) and bile acids. Too much cholesterol, however, can damage your arteries and heart. So, although the liver makes cholesterol and passes it into the blood, it also takes cholesterol from the blood stream.

Though some of the cholesterol in the liver is made into bile acids, some passes into the bile as "free" cholesterol, only about 40% of which is reabsorbed by the intestine. The remaining 60% is passed out of the body. The liver also makes a carrier substance which collects excess cholesterol from the tissues of the body and brings it back to the liver for processing. The right balance of cholesterol in the body is needed for you to keep well, and the liver is an essential controller of this.

Cholesterol is a fat-like substance found in all animal cells. It is needed to make hormones and bile acids. Too much can damage your heart and arteries. Amount in your bloodstream is regulated by liver.

It's a processor

The liver is a processor of blood components. When red blood cells are old and require removing from the bloodstream, they are broken down in the spleen. This process releases haemoglobin, the red, oxygen-carrying chemical which is converted to bilirubin, a yellowish-green pigment, and carried in the bloodstream to the liver. There it is modified chemically to another type of bilirubin (conjugated bilirubin), which can then be passed down the bile ducts and eventually eliminated from the body.

When you take drugs as part of medical treatment, your liver often plays an important part in converting these to harmless products that can be safely disposed of by the kidneys or the liver itself. Paracetamol, a very effective and useful painkiller, is an example of a drug that is dealt with in this way.

Bilirubin is a yellow pigment formed from blood wastes; in many liver diseases it accumulates in the blood and causes jaundice.

It's a sink

The liver is a sink which allows the body to get rid of unwanted excess chemicals such as bilirubin, cholesterol, and various drugs through the bile.

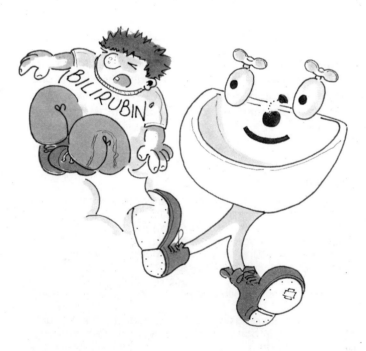

And a store

The liver is a store for energy such as the carbohydrate, glycogen, which is converted to sugar in case your body runs short of energy. It is also a store for vitamin B12 which helps the marrow to make blood properly.

What upsets the liver:
- **Alcohol**
- **Infections**
- **Drugs**
- **Herbs**
- **Cancer**
- **Auto-immune diseases**
- **Diabetes**

What can make the liver go wrong?

There are several things that are known to stop the liver working properly.

Alcohol

Drinking too much alcohol causes liver disease and damages the liver.

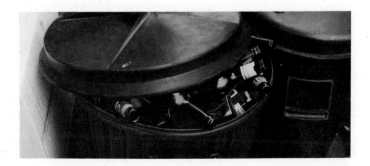

Infections

Viral infections such as hepatitis, glandular fever, and yellow fever can cause severe liver damage and sometimes lead to long term ill health.

Drugs and herbs

Drugs (and some herbs!) can cause liver damage. This is well known and predictable with overdoses of paracetamol or drinking too much comfrey tea, but it may also be an unusual, personal reaction as with the anaesthetic gas halothane or heavy tranquillisers such as chlorpromazine.

Cancer

Cancer can affect the liver either by spreading to the liver from elsewhere or by a tumour arising in the liver itself.

Auto-immune diseases

The liver can be damaged by curious diseases in which the body reacts against itself (so-called auto-immune diseases). Examples of these are chronic active hepatitis and primary biliary cirrhosis. After a liver transplant, a similar process can destroy the new grafted liver.

Other diseases

The liver may be involved in diseases, such as diabetes, that mainly affect other parts of the body. Sometimes this can be severe as with cirrhosis or liver abscesses seen in ulcerative colitis.

Effect of a damaged liver

When the liver is severely damaged other parts of the body can be affected, especially the spleen. Because high pressure builds up in the portal vein in patients with cirrhosis, their spleen becomes swollen. It may then become overactive and destroy too much blood instead of just the old cells that needed removing.

What the pancreas does

The pancreas has two different jobs. It is best known as the gland that makes insulin, which is passed directly into the bloodstream and is needed to control the way the body uses sugars. The pancreas's second job is to make a digestive juice which it sends down the pancreatic duct to the intestine. This juice contains alkali to neutralise the acid made in the stomach, so helping to prevent ulcers forming in the duodenum. It also contains enzymes which digest the fat, carbohydrate, and protein in our food so that they can be properly absorbed.

Although the insulin-making part of the pancreas is mixed up with the part that makes pancreatic juice, they are quite separate in the way that they work.

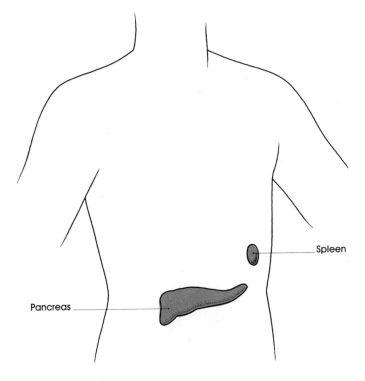

Spleen

Pancreas

The pancreas and spleen.

What the spleen does

The spleen is useful but not absolutely essential. It is part of the body's immune defence system against infection and is also a blood filter. According to legend, Greek athletes sometimes had it removed before races to get a slightly better turn of speed, which sounds a pretty desperate measure.

In adults, the spleen sorts out the old blood cells as they need to be replaced by new ones from the bone marrow. The old cells are broken up so that their components can be re-used — one of the many jobs done by the liver. If your spleen has to be removed then you are not fully protected from certain bacterial infections and may need to be given permanent treatment with penicillin.

2 What can go wrong with the liver?

Jaundice

The word jaundice means "yellowness". If your skin and the whites of your eyes become yellow this is an important clue that there is liver disease. Usually the cause is a build up of the pigment bilirubin in the blood. This stains most of the body tissues and can easily be seen in the whites of the eyes and in a white person's skin. There are, however, one or two other fascinating but rare causes of yellowness — such as eating too many carrots.

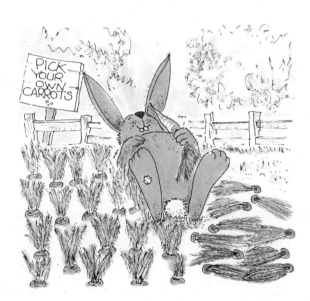

Bilirubin

Normal blood fluid (plasma) always contains a little bilirubin so that when it is separated from the cells in blood it looks pale yellow. The red colour of whole blood comes from a substance called haemoglobin in blood cells. Haemoglobin has the job of carrying oxygen from the lungs around the body. When blood cells age and break down, the red haemoglobin is released and changes to yellow bilirubin.

Bilirubin travels around in the blood stream to the liver where it is processed and joins with another substance to form conjugated bilirubin. Conjugated bilirubin dissolves very easily in water and can be converted quickly by the liver into bile. When bile is very concentrated the bilirubin colours it vividly so that it looks like golden treacle. After the bile has travelled down the ducts to the intestine, bilirubin is changed again to give the brown colour to stools.

Different things can go wrong with this system and cause jaundice.

When the balance is disturbed

Blood may be broken down too quickly so that a normal liver, working flat out, cannot clear the bilirubin as quickly as it is made from haemoglobin. If you have this problem you will usually become anaemic, with a low number of red blood cells in the bloodstream (and peculiarly shaped red cells). This can happen in some inherited illnesses and as a side effect of certain drug treatments.

Gilbert's syndrome

The liver needs to change free bilirubin into conjugated bilirubin before it can be passed by the bile and intestine out of the body. In some otherwise quite healthy people, the liver cannot conjugate bilirubin very well. This disorder is called Gilbert's syndrome, — it is not a serious disease but a fairly harmless condition that causes jaundice and affects more than 1% of the whole population. Gilbert's syndrome is usually diagnosed after episodes of jaundice and it is also often highlighted by other illnesses.

One **Scottish** professional **footballer** developed mild viral disease that affected his liver (hepatitis). He recovered well, but later had more jaundice despite feeling perfectly fit. He and his club were very anxious in case he might have permanent liver damage which could affect his play. Tests showed that his liver looked quite normal under the microscope but that he had Gilbert's syndrome. He was reassured, and also told to explain the diagnosis to any doctor treating him in the future so that his liver did not come under unfair suspicion again.

Liver damage or Inflammation

When the liver is seriously inflamed or damaged, bilirubin builds up in the blood and reaches levels that cause a person to look yellow. This type of jaundice happens when liver cells cannot conjugate bilirubin properly (and thereby eliminate it from the body) and is seen in the illnesses cirrhosis and hepatitis.

No escape

Even when the liver cells are working well to make conjugated bilirubin, the bilirubin may not be able to escape in the bile. This can happen when the tiny branches of the bile ducts in the liver are damaged or when the larger bile ducts are blocked. Blockage can be caused by gallstones in the bile duct, by cancer in the pancreas (which squeezes the common bile duct), or by narrowing of the bile duct itself for other reasons. If the conjugated bilirubin has no escape route, the stools go pale and bilirubin is passed out in urine, which becomes very dark as a result.

Some other causes

Though most of the causes of jaundice can be explained in the ways described, other problems are important too. For example, acute inflammation of the gallbladder may cause jaundice even when the bile ducts do not seem to be blocked. Also, patients who have other serious illnesses such as heart failure can become jaundiced, possibly because the blood flow to the liver is poor.

Fluid

In chronic (long term) liver damage fluid may collect in the body, especially in the abdomen. This is partly because the pressure in the veins to the liver is high, forcing fluid out, and partly because the liver does not make enough protein to keep the general circulation working properly. Also there is a mysterious connection between the diseased liver and the kidneys which do not filter as well as they ought and keep too much water and salt in the body.

There may be such small amounts of fluid that they can barely be found. On the other hand, sometimes there is so much that the belly looks like a twin pregnancy.

The skin can be affected too, giving a puffy face and swollen ankles.

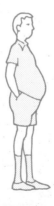

Bleeding

If your liver is diseased your blood may not clot properly because the liver makes a whole family of proteins which stop bleeding. Sometimes an injection of vitamin K will stimulate the liver to make one of these proteins to help your blood to clot.

Another reason that bleeding may happen is because of too much pressure in the veins of the liver. This can make the spleen swollen and work harder than it should. The spleen may then break down too many of the blood particles called platelets, which are also needed to form blood clots.

Bruises

You can tell that your blood is not clotting properly if your skin bruises. Inside your body very serious and life-threatening bleeding can occur. People with liver disease often get ulcers in the duodenum (the small intestine) which may bleed readily. They also get big veins at the bottom of the oesophagus or gullet (where food passes through to the stomach) which are fragile and can bleed torrentially.

Anaemia

If a person bleeds internally the body may run short of blood and of iron, which is needed to make blood, and this leads to anaemia. This is worsened if the person has not been eating properly and has run short of B vitamins.

One of the interesting things that alcohol does to the body is to prevent the bone marrow making blood properly. So if an alcoholic with liver disease just gives up drinking this may be enough to improve anaemia.

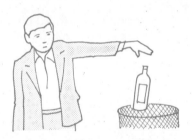

Itch and diarrhoea

The liver makes bile acids to help digest fats. If the liver is diseased or the bile flow is blocked then not enough bile acid gets into the intestine, fat is not absorbed well, and a peculiar diarrhoea follows. The stools are bulky and yellow, and — even more noticeable — they tend to be smelly and difficult to flush away.

The bile acid which did not get into the intestine may collect in the liver and damage cells there. It may also spill over into the bloodstream. It is thought that bile acids in the blood and in the skin may cause the itching, which is common in some types of liver disease and when the bile ducts are blocked.

Mental problems

People with severe liver disease have trouble thinking. This is because poisonous breakdown products of protein from the diet and from the body itself are not processed normally. In addition, the brain becomes more sensitive, so that even small doses of normally harmless drugs or alcohol may cause serious problems.

Depression and confusion

Sometimes the person with liver disease becomes lethargic and depressed. But over a long time confusion and poor memory may be more serious problems. This is not always obvious and people learn to cover it up to avoid embarrassment.

The test, which you can do yourself, is to draw a five-pointed star without taking the pen off the paper. Another test is to join in order 25 numbered dots scattered over a page as quickly as possible. The five-pointed star should be recognisable as a star to other people and the "dottogram" should be completed in about half a minute.

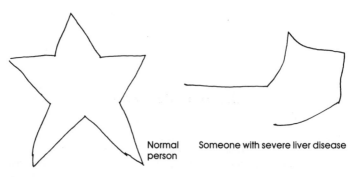

Normal person

Someone with severe liver disease

Coma

When the liver damage is very serious a coma can develop which deepens and causes the breathing to stop and death. As the coma deepens the person may become irritable and have fits. These fits are very difficult to treat because doctors have to give high doses of sedative drugs, which are dangerous for someone already in coma.

3 What can go wrong with the pancreas?

If your pancreas doesn't make insulin and pass it into the blood stream, you can develop diabetes. But there are other serious diseases of the pancreas, of which the most important are inflammation, or pancreatitis, cystic fibrosis, and cancer.

Inflammation of the pancreas

The pancreas can become inflamed. That means that it swells, causes pain, and may not work effectively. This can happen suddenly — acute pancreatitis — but settle down completely in a short time, or it may slowly get worse — chronic pancreatitis. If this happens the tissues and cells will fail to do their job of producing the enzymes that help your digestion.

Acute pancreatitis

A short, sudden attack of pain is often caused by gallstones passing down the bile duct. If this happens again and again, the gallbladder can be removed and the bile duct cleared of stones — and that should clear it.

Sometimes alcohol is the cause, usually in someone who is a heavy drinker. But the attack may not particularly be related to a binge. Acute pancreatitis is painful, and you usually go to hospital where you are given strong painkillers and treated for any complications.

25

Chronic pancreatitis

Chronic — or persistent — pancreatitis is seen in people who are alcoholics, but it can occur for no clear reason. The pain in the abdomen and the backache may be so bad that you drink even more alcohol to try to deaden it. People with painful chronic pancreatitis sometimes become addicted to narcotic drugs used for pain relief, and suicides have also occurred. Because digestive enzymes are not produced you lose weight and have diarrhoea.

It is possible to take tablets or capsules with food to help your digestion. In the worst types of chronic pancreatitis part or all of the pancreas can be removed and this should cure the symptoms. However, that will cause other problems like diabetes and an even worse shortage of digestive enzymes. Though quite a few people die after this operation, people are usually so very unwell, and their life is such a torment, that they are willing to take the risk of operation to improve their quality of life.

Cancer

About 5000 people each year in Britain develop cancer of the pancreas and it is gradually getting commoner. Because it is very difficult to diagnose this cancer early enough to cure it or even to treat it at all, it is almost always a fatal disease. We do not yet know how we can prevent this cancer of the pancreas from developing.

Pancreas disorders
- **Diabetes (insulin imbalance)**
- **Acute pancreatitis (gallstones and alcohol)**
- **Chronic pancreatitis (usually alcohol)**
- **Cancer (getting commoner)**

4 What can go wrong with the gallbladder and bile ducts?

Gallstone disease

The main thing that can go wrong with your gallbladder is that you might develop gallstones. These can also develop in the bile ducts. In the gallbladder stones can cause inflammation — acute cholecystitis — or severe pains which are often right-sided and spread to your back (biliary colic). Moving into the bile duct, gallstones may block the bile, causing obstructive jaundice or an attack of acute pancreatitis. Cancer of the gallbladder is uncommon.

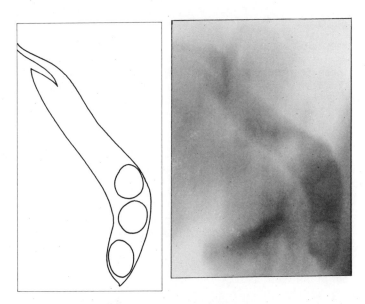

The x-ray film of the gallbladder shows several large stones.

Stones in bile ducts

Sometimes stones form in the bile ducts themselves, caused for instance, by a surgical stitch after an operation, or in Eastern countries by parasitic worms.

If damaged, the bile duct may be too narrow for the bile to flow. This is called a stricture and may cause jaundice and allow infections to spread back to the liver.

Cancer of bile ducts

Cancer of the bile ducts, which is not at all common, also blocks the flow of bile. This can be very difficult indeed to diagnose, especially if the cancer is in the smaller bile ducts.

How bile is made

Bile Acids

Bile acids are the substances in the bile which help to absorb fat. The liver sends bile acids down the bile ducts continuously. These acids form tiny clusters of particles called micelles which dissolve completely in water. They cannot be seen even with the most powerful microscope using light, but only with the electron microscope, which allows very small structures to be examined.

Two paths

The bile acids can go two ways. They can pass down the whole system of bile ducts and enter the intestine directly. Or they can go into the gallbladder instead where they are stored and concentrated until you eat a meal. Then the gallbladder contracts to send a flood of bile into the duodenum (small intestine).

Fat in the diet

The fat that you eat cannot be fully digested or absorbed into your body until the bile acids make it dissolvable in water. This is called emulsifying. When fat is emulsified the digestive enzymes from the pancreas break the food down into simple fragments which are readily absorbed. The bile acids are absorbed separately and almost completely so that little is excreted from your body.

The gallbladder at work

The gallbladder will contract about twice during a meal, so that it contracts about half a dozen times a day. Overnight after supper the gallbladder will gradually fill up with concentrated bile ready and waiting for the breakfast egg and bacon, buttered toast, and the milk on the cornflakes and in the tea.

It does not need to do this because if your gallbladder has been removed you can still enjoy a well digested breakfast too.

Horses, pigeons, and rats are some of the animals that do quite well without a gallbladder.

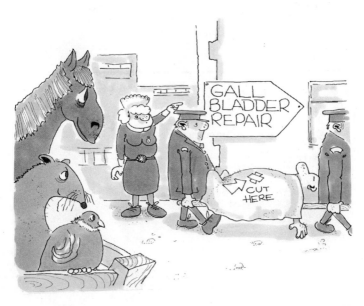

What's in the bile?

The bile contains a lot of other things, not just bile acids. There are proteins, bicarbonate, calcium salts, conjugated bilirubin, and, most importantly, cholesterol.

Cholesterol

Because the liver sends a lot of cholesterol into the bile it has to have a special system to keep the cholesterol mixed in with the bile. In the bloodstream cholesterol is carried by special proteins, but bile has very little protein, so a different method is needed.

Lecithin

The liver makes a substance lecithin — one of a category rich in phosphorus called phospholipids. Before passing into the bile, the lecithin and the cholesterol join together to form minute bubbles which quickly disappear by joining up with the clumps of bile acids. These bubbles are so tiny and disappear so quickly that research workers, who have been studying bile for more than 20 years, overlooked their importance until recently.

Gallstones are made of:
- **Cholesterol**
- **Bilirubin**
- **Calcium salts — uncommon**

---

5 How gallstones form

In Western societies most gallstones are mainly made of cholesterol. Some gallstones are made purely of bilirubin — the yellow-green pigment — or, even more rarely of calcium salts. Even if there is some bilirubin or calcium salts, most of the gallstone is usually made up of cholesterol.

A delicate balance

The bile in your body is in a delicate balance because even in normal people at certain times there is more cholesterol than will dissolve in the bile solution. This can happen overnight. And if you deliberately do not eat for a long time it makes it worse.

It takes more than cholesterol

But this excess cholesterol is not enough to cause gallstones on its own. There has to be some trigger factor which starts off the process of forming crystals.

It is thought that in the bile of people who have gallstones there are elements that promote crystallisation. These might be proteins which are found in the mucus (slime) which the gallbladder produces in small amounts. These encourage the cholesterol to form particles like tiny solid crystals.

Crystals

These crystals probably start to form from the bubbles made up of the phospholipid, lecithin and cholesterol, and they become too large to remain dissolved in the bile. The crystals grow by making more cholesterol come out of the bile solution on the surface.

Although these elements that promote crystallisation are in the bile of healthy people too, they are blocked, probably by other proteins, from forming crystals.

Once the crystals start to form they probably don't stop or reverse, so that the stones tend to increase in number and size and rarely disappear on their own.

Bilirubin

The bilirubin in bile dissolves very easily, and if left alone would never cause problems. However, bilirubin can be broken down by an enzyme — a protein which causes a chemical reaction — which is found in the bile tube, and which is also found in certain bacteria and worms that can infect the bile. When this happens the free bilirubin may join with the cholesterol to make mixed stones. Or it may form pigment stones on its own, or with calcium. Stones which contain only calcium are not common, though in Japan in the past, when very few Japanese had gallstones, calcium stones were the most common. This sort of mineral stone is much more often seen in the organs and ducts that pass urine.

Sorts of stones

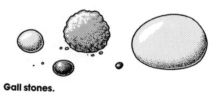

Gall stones.

The various sorts of gallstones are very different. Cholesterol stones are yellow and greasy. Pigment stones are black and hard or brown and crumbly. The size can vary too — from pinheads that you can hardly see, through gravel, to large "rocks" which can be several centimetres (1 to 2″) across. The largest gallstones can completely fill the gallbladder so that there is no room left for bile. The result is as if you had no gallbladder at all. This is very uncommon. The average size is about 1 to 2 centimetres (about ½″) across.

Of course, all you need to cause trouble is one gallstone, but there is usually more than one. And, several thousand have been found on some people! When several large gallstones are in the gallbladder together they tend to flatten out where they touch.

Normally stones form in the gallbladder itself when a stagnant pool of bile sits for some time. But they can move into the bile ducts and get stuck there. Sometimes gallstones actually form in the bile duct first, but this doesn't happen often.

6 Who gets gallstones?

We can find out how common gallstones are in different groups of people or different countries. This is possible by gathering information from examinations that have been carried out on people who have died and by examining people's gallbladders by a technique called ultrasound or by X rays.

Race and country

Race is very important. The American Indians who live in the southwestern United States hold the world record for getting gallstones. Half the women in these tribes have gallstones by the time they are 30. The Hispanic North Americans also have a lot of gallstones. White people in the USA have a moderate number, but black people in the USA have fewer.

This is the best information we have about gallstones in different races. But though these groups of people live in the same country, they live under different conditions of life so that their environment probably is important as well as heredity.

In general, in industrialised and developed countries, such as Sweden, Czechoslovakia, and the United Kingdom, more people have gallstones than in less developed countries, such as many of the African states.

VERY HIGH	HIGH	MODERATE	LOW
North American Indians	USA whites	USA blacks	Greece
Chile	Great Britain	Japan	Egypt
Sweden	Norway	Singapore	Zambia
Czechoslovakia	Australia		Uganda
Mexican Americans	Italy		Nigeria

Gall stones in different countries and races.

An unusual case

Japan is a very interesting country because at the turn of the century gallstones were not common at all, and when they did occur they were mainly made of mineral and pigment. Now that Japan has adopted a Western lifestyle and diet, gallstones have become more frequent. And, they are now usually composed of cholesterol, like the ones that develop in the West.

Britain

Gallstones are very common in Britain. We know, too, that they have become more common over the past 35 years in all age groups. Before the mid-1950s the information is not so reliable, but probably between the beginning of the 20th century and the second world war the numbers of people who developed gallstones did not change much. Most of the information is about white Britons, so that changes in population through immigration would not have had much effect.

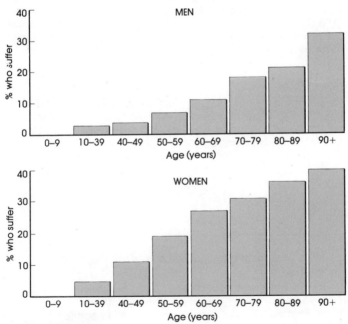

Gall stones in Britain.

Age

Age is a key factor in developing gallstones. Although it is possible to be born with gallstones (which can now be diagnosed in the fetus inside the mother!) this is mercifully exceptionally rare. Very little gallstone disease is seen until after puberty. Thereafter, a gradual increase with age occurs so that the chance that people in their 90s and older will have gallstones is as high as one in three. So even if nothing else changed, because the general population is getting older gallstones will be a more frequent problem than before.

Female sex

Being a woman is risky for getting gallstones. At every age women have more gallstones than men, but this evens up later in life in the elderly. The foolish notion that middle aged women are more prone to gallstones is still common, despite evidence in many surveys that old women (and men) have more.

Pregnancy

Pregnancy is of course a female prerogative, and it is important to know that women who have had more than two full length pregnancies have an increased risk of gallstones. This might be ammunition for the family planners.

Important factors for gallstone disease
- **Race**
- **Industrialised countries**
- **Age**
- **Female sex**
- **Obesity**
- **Drugs**
- **Anaemia**

Does the "pill" cause gallstones?

The oral contraceptive pill *does not* cause gallstones. At first there was some confusion because of misleading studies published in the 1970s. But now more recent studies show that in this respect the pill is blameless.

Overweight

Being excessively overweight makes people more likely to get gallstones.

You can easily work out whether you are too fat.

Body Mass Index

You take your height in metres and multiply it by itself. Then take that number and divide it into your weight in kilograms. This gives you what is called the Body Mass Index.

The ideal for women is 19 to 24, and for men 20 to 25. If your number is over 30, you are obese — and this is a risk to your health. If your number is over 40, life will be significantly shorter.

> I am 1.76 metres tall and weigh 77.5 kilograms, so my Body Mass Index is 25. This confirms my opinion that I am ideal — and my colleagues' opinion that I am on the verge of not being so!

Losing weight

Though being severely overweight may cause gallstones, if a person who is very overweight loses a lot of weight quickly this can also cause gallstones. Sometimes operations are performed to help people who are very fat to lose weight, and so it may be necessary to give them drugs to stop them from getting gallstones while the weight is falling. The new slim individual at the end of the process has an improved chance of avoiding gallstones.

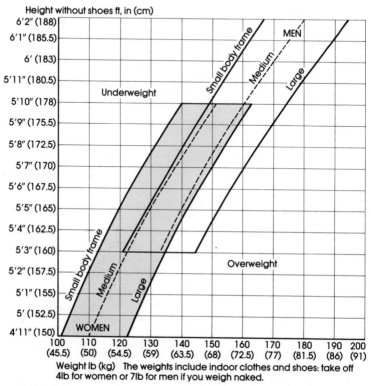

Height without shoes ft, in (cm)

Weight lb (kg) The weights include indoor clothes and shoes: take off 4lb for women or 7lb for men if you weigh naked.

Weight chart.

Diet

Diet has been blamed for most of life's ills, but no particular part of our diet can be convincingly blamed for causing gallstones. Cholesterol, fat, protein, and carbohydrates have all been studied and were found not to be important. It has been suggested that diets with a lot of roughage — that is, food with lots of indigestible fibre — such as eaten in rural Africa, might prevent stones forming, but the case is not strong. Vegetarians, however, do seem to be protected from gallstones. Moderate quantities of alcohol improve the solubility of cholesterol in bile, and it would be very nice to think that this would be beneficial in stopping stones forming.

Drugs

Drugs which affect cholesterol in the body are important causes of changes in bile. One group of drugs works by making the liver push cholesterol out of the body and into the bile, and has caused more cholesterol gallstones to form. Clofibrate (Atromid S) is one of these drugs, and it is thought that the closely related drugs, gemfibrozil and bezafibrate, also may cause stones. The other sorts of drugs used to clear cholesterol such as cholestyramine (Questran) do not seem to carry this risk. No other drugs have been convincingly shown to be important in causing gallstones.

Anaemia

Haemolytic anaemia, in which the blood is broken down too quickly, causes a larger amount of bilirubin than normal in the liver for passage into the bile. For some reason this causes an excess of gallstones which are often rich in pigment. This is one of the important causes of gallstones in children.

Gallstones are common

Gallstones can run in families, but they are so common in the whole community that it is not usually possible to blame parents rather than life in general. Knowing what we do about how often stones develop and how precarious the chemical balance of bile is, it would be a more realistic question to ask why we don't all get gallstones.

7 How do gallstones show up?

Sometimes there are no symptoms

From studies of populations we know that most gallstones are silent — don't cause any symptoms — and never seem to cause any problems. For instance, in the small town of Sirmione in Italy two thirds of the adults were examined. Over three quarters of the people who had gallstones did not have any symptoms. We also have evidence from other surveys to confirm this impression, so we have to accept that the majority of gallstones do not cause symptoms. This is very important because they may be blamed unfairly for symptoms which have other explanations.

When there are symptoms

When definite diseases are caused by gallstones several patterns can be recognised.

Biliary colic

Biliary colic is a severe pain in the upper abdomen which starts at any time, and it can wake you up at night. It may be worse on the right side, and spread through to your back or go all round in a band. It generally lasts hours before going away and can cause you to vomit. You often need to see the doctor to get relief, and the pain tends to keep coming back at intervals.

Obstructive jaundice

Obstructive jaundice can occur when the flow of bile is blocked by a gallstone in the duct. It is often painful and you go yellow and then a green shade if you are not treated. You must find out what is wrong quickly to avoid damaging your liver. This may be difficult because the jaundice may be caused by other problems even if you have gallstones.

Acute cholecystitis

Acute cholecystitis is a condition in which the gallbladder is inflamed. It's usually thought to happen when a gallstone gets stuck in the narrow entrance to the gallbladder. This may develop suddenly or gradually over a few days. You feel pain and tenderness in the upper right abdomen and have a fever. If the infection continues the whole gallbladder can become full of pus, like an abscess.

Acute pancreatitis

Acute pancreatitis — a sudden, short attack of pain — can be caused by gallstones. Alcohol is another common cause. The sex war rears its head here since a man with acute pancreatitis tends to be suspected of heavy drinking, whereas a woman who has more than one episode of acute pancreatitis is considered to have gallstones until proved otherwise. It is probably caused by small stones passing down the ducts into the intestine, which inflame the opening into the small intestine and the pancreatic duct.

Peculiar tummies

Although it has been thought that indigestion caused by fats, and other complaints about digestion, can be related to gallstones, this is untrue.

These complaints may actually get worse if the gallbladder is mistakenly removed. Another cause can be discovered for some of these symptoms. But for many no cause can be found and those people just have to come to terms with the fact that their "tummies are peculiar".

8 How do you find gallstones?

Ultrasound

Most gallstones are found in the gallbladder and are big enough to be found very easily. Nowadays the most useful test for finding gallstones is ultrasound, in which echoes which cannot be heard by human ears are bounced off your insides. A sound picture is shown on a screen and photographs can be taken of this. It's pretty difficult for anyone to make head or tail of these pictures unless they were present at the test.

Gallstones block the passage of soundwaves through them and throw a sound shadow behind. Gallstones also move about in the gallbladder when you alter your position. The ultrasound test is 98% reliable, which is medical perfection, because doctors are always suspicious of anything which claims to be totally right!

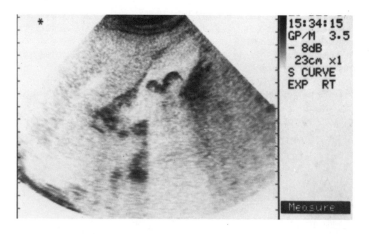

Oral cholecystogram

An older test which can also be used is the oral cholecystogram. In this test you take tablets of an iodine compound which your body absorbs and passes into the bile where it is concentrated in the gallbladder. X rays are taken and the stones show as gaps in the iodine compound. This test has drawbacks because it requires preparation, you must not be sensitive to iodine, and the gallbladder may not oblige by concentrating the dye. These days doctors tend to use it only when other tests have given no clear answer.

Other tests

About one in 10 gallstones can be seen on an X ray of the abdomen. But this must usually be confirmed by an ultrasound test or oral cholecystography to avoid mistakes.

When you are ill with acute cholecystitis the gallbladder stops working, and this can be shown by a radioisotope test if it is carried out quickly. Again, some other test has to confirm that there are gallstones there before it is thought certain that stones are present. If the isotope test proves that the gallbladder is still working, then the diagnosis of acute cholecystitis was wrong and the doctor has to think again.

If there are stones in the bile duct they may not be easy to see. Ultrasound misses about half of them but it may show that the bile ducts have widened.

Injecting dye

Another technique, injecting iodine X ray contrast dye, may give better pictures. This technique (called endoscopy) is usually done by the patient swallowing a flexible fibreoptic instrument which allows the stomach and duodenum to be seen. This instrument is steered to the duodenum, and a plastic tube is passed down an internal channel in the instrument and dye is squirted into the bile and pancreatic ducts to make X ray pictures.

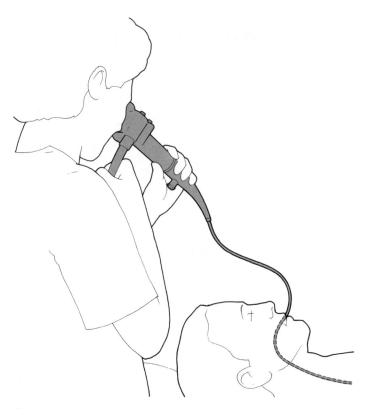

Endoscopy.

Another method is to stick a long fine needle through the skin and across the liver into the top end of the bile ducts to inject dye this way. If you are not bright yellow from jaundice the X ray dye can sometimes be given by drip into a vein in the arm. Then when the liver has cleared the dye into the bile ducts X rays can be taken.

Blood tests

Blood tests are not a lot of help in diagnosing gallstones.

Does the gallbladder get diseased without Stones?

Generally doctors are not very happy about blaming the gallbladder for any symptoms if no stones can be found in it. There are exceptions. One is when there are tiny stones in the gallbladder that do not show up on ultrasound or *X* ray tests. Another is that in patients who are gravely ill for other reasons a curious infection which fills the gallbladder with gas can happen. With this dramatic exception, a gallbladder without stones in it is probably best left alone.

When do gallstones matter?

Most gallstones never cause health problems. So it is important to decide which ones are worth bothering about.

Finding gallstones unexpectedly

Sometimes gallstones are found by chance. When *X* rays are taken after a back injury the ring shadow of a chalky stone may be found.

Sometimes gallstones break inside and these cracks fill with gas and show three lines spreading from the centre of the stones — the Mercedes-Benz sign.

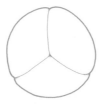

Sometimes ultrasound tests that are carried out to measure the size of arteries or for other reasons may pick up gallstones. Operations on the belly for other problems may turn up gallstones too.

In all of these cases the stones are usually best left alone.

When gallstones cause symptoms

Once gallstones do cause definite symptoms they tend to go on doing so, and the problems may get worse and worse. A person who has had cholecystitis — acute inflamation of the gallbladder — jaundice, or more than one attack of colic or pancreatitis needs treatment.

If stones are found in the bile duct, then it is very important to clear them because they can cause serious illness and even death. On the other hand, stones that stay only in the gallbladder rarely cause anyone to die, so a decision about your treatment is made on the basis of your symptoms.

For instance, in about 5000 postmortem examinations carried out in Dundee hospitals from 1974 to 1983, there were only 22 deaths from gallbladder stones, but there were also 22 deaths after the removal of the gallbladder, which is regarded as a very safe operation!

9 How do you treat gallstones?

Treatment for pain

When you have severe pain from gallstones, then an injection is given of an opium-type drug, such as pethidine. Because these powerful painkillers usually cause nausea, you often get another injection to keep you from getting sick.

Because the pain of gallstone colic is linked to muscle spasm, anti-spasm drugs have been tried too. Injection of the drug atropine, or a similar drug, should help the pain. But it doesn't always do the job.

Prostaglandins

Recently it has been suggested that inflammation of the gallbladder and bile ducts is directly caused by substances named prostaglandins, which are like hormones. Powerful drugs are available to counteract prostaglandins, such as diclofenac, which has been tested and found to work. Giving drugs like this avoids the need for possibly repeated injections of opiates which are potentially addictive. Also it may be possible for the doctor to leave you with a supply of the drug and a syringe to use in case of need.

Treating the pain
- **Pethidine**
- **Atropine**
- **Diclofenac**

Surgery for gallstones

The operation to remove the gallbladder for stones — cholecystectomy — had its 100th birthday in 1982 and it is still going strong. This is still the best treatment for most gallstones.

How the operation is done

The surgeon makes either a diagonal cut in the upper right side of the abdomen, or a vertical cut near the centre of the upper abdomen. The muscles are moved aside or split or cut across, and the lining of the inside of the abdomen is opened. The gallbladder is found under the liver, and the blood supply to the gallbladder is stopped. The gallbladder is removed with the stones inside.

The surgeon takes great care not to leave a long cystic duct behind, and not to cut the cystic ducts so short that the common bile duct, which takes bile from the liver to the small intestine is damaged.

The ill health suffered by Sir Anthony Eden because of gallstones and a damaged bile duct in the 1950s may have led to some of the bad decision-making responsible for the Suez crisis.

Bile ducts are checked for stones

Nowadays surgeons are very careful to examine the bile ducts and make sure there are no stones here, because otherwise there will be more problems. They do this by putting a plastic tube into the cut end of the cystic duct and injecting iodine contrast dye into the bile ducts before X rays are made.

Another test is to pass a flexible fine instrument called a fibreoptic choledochoscope or a rigid "gas pipe" choledochoscope into the bile duct and look to make sure the passages are clear.

If there are stones in the bile duct they can be removed either by cutting a small hole in the bile duct or by catching the stones in a wire basket that is passed through the choledochoscope. If the bile duct has to be cleared of stones like this, a drain shaped like the letter "T" is placed with the cross-piece in the bile duct. The long arm is brought out through the skin and allowed to syphon off the bile. About seven or 10 days after the operation X-ray contrast dye is injected to make sure there are no other stones left. If the test shows that the duct is clear the T-tube drain is removed simply by pulling on the long end until it comes out. It sounds horrible but it does work, and the hole in the bile duct does seal off.

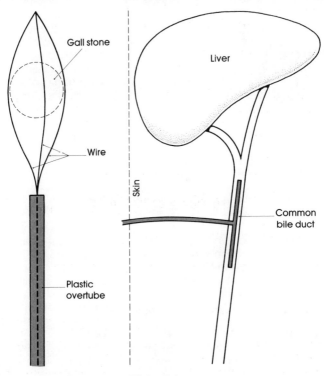

Dormia basket.

T-tube drain.

Always a risk

The results for cholecystectomy have got better and better over the years, but no surgical treatment is without risk. One recent example was the death of the world famous multimillionaire artist Andy Warhol after a simple gallbladder operation when he was apparently in good health.

Nowadays less than 1 in 100 people die after the procedure, and for anyone who is fit and young or middle aged this should be more like 1 in 1000. The overall results reflect the fact that many of the operations have to be carried out on elderly people who also have other health problems.

Do people get cured?

After the gallbladder is removed six out of every 10 people are completely cured of serious symptoms. Two out of every 10 are improved but not completely cured. This leaves about 1 out of every 10 who is not helped, and an even more puzzling 1 out of 10 who say they are worse! These two groups sometimes have stones in the bile tubes either because they were left behind or because more formed. Some of the people have further tests and are found to have different problems. Most remain something of a mystery.

Fashions in treatment

There are fashions in surgical treatment as with everything else. Women with gallstones are more likely to have operations than men, perhaps because they complain to the doctor more than men do, or maybe because doctors expect them to have gallstone problems more often. Since the second world war cholecystectomy has been performed more often in many countries including Britain. It is the commonest abdominal operation in Britain now, beating even operations to remove the appendix. In Sweden the trend has been the other way, with fewer and fewer operations, even though gallstones are still very common there.

Britain and other countries

Also, where you live makes a difference as to how likely you are to get an operation. In Britain and Spain about 1 out of 7 to 1 out of 10 patients with gallstones get surgery. But in the USA and Italy it's 1 out of three.

It is thought that the figure for Britain is about right and that the Americans do too many operations. This may reflect that there are many more surgeons in North America, and that (under their health care system) they have to operate if they want to earn any money.

It seems likely that the number of gallstone operations in Britain will not increase and it may actually decrease in future.

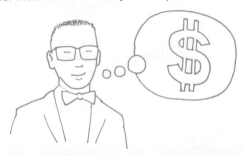

Is diet treatment useful for gallstones?

The short answer to whether a special diet is good for gallstones is — not very. Doctors used to think that since a contraction of the gallbladder causes a flood of bile into the intestine, which helps to digest fats, then restricting fat in the diet would avoid a spasm of the gallbladder and colic.

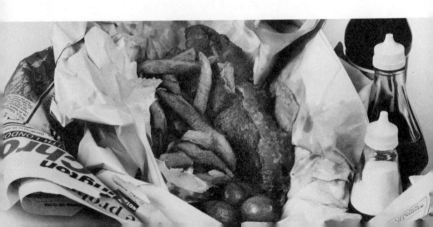

Eat what you like

Unfortunately, it does not work out like that. Almost any food or drink, including just a glass of water, will make the gallbladder contract, and it is hardly practical to recommend complete starvation to control symptoms! In practice, most people with gallstones do not find that a change to their diet affects their symptoms. So there is not much point in a general recommendation of low fat diet.

Occasionally there is a clear link between what a person eats and the symptoms. For example, one of my patients had no trouble as long as he avoided fried eggs for breakfast. But unless there is a convincing connection between particular foods and colic, it is not worth while interfering with the diet.

Dissolving gallstones

When doctors realised that the cholesterol in bile was important for gallstone disease, a search started for drugs which could be taken safely by mouth to reduce cholesterol in the bile and so encourage gallstones to dissolve back into bile.

This treatment is only suitable for certain people. The two drugs most commonly used are both bile acids. One is called chenodeoxycholic acid. The other is ursodeoxycholic acid.

Both of these bile acids will dissolve cholesterol stones that are smaller than 15 mm (about ½″) in diameter if the stones do not contain much calcium and are either in a gallbladder which is working normally or in bile ducts which are not blocked.

Big doses of chenodeoxycholic acid are needed, but this often causes diarrhoea. The diarrhoea can be helped by taking a lower dose, but some of the effectiveness is lost. Rather smaller doses are used with ursodeoxycholic acid, which seems to be pretty free of side effects.

You take this treatment continuously, and your gallbladder is tested every six months or so by ultrasound or oral cholecystography to see whether stones have got smaller or gone altogether. To prove complete success you must have two negative tests — one of which at least should be ultrasound. Generally there is some sign of improvement at six months, but if the stones do not change at all after two years the treatment is stopped.

About one third to a half of patients selected for this treatment will have their stones completely dissolved.

Who has this treatment?

Dissolving stones can be useful where an operation is not desirable.

A medical student in his final year developed gallstone disease and wanted to take his exams without any delay so that he could take the medical jobs already arranged. He had several gallbladder stones up to about 10 mm (less than ½") in diameter. After taking chenodeoxycholic acid for six months the stones were smaller, and after a year they had completely gone. He finished his studies and had no further problems.

A fascinating feature of bile acid treatment is that people have immediate relief of symptoms. A third have no more pain and a third are greatly improved even before the gallstones start to dissolve.

Will they come back?

The big drawback of dissolving stones without removing the gallbladder is that they can recur. They recur in about 10% of people after one year, in 20% at two years, and in 35% at 3½ years, with no more problems after that. No really good way of preventing this happening is known.

Perhaps if people kept taking bile acids it would stop more stones forming — but this would mean a life sentence of drug treatment. The other plan is either to wait for more symptoms or to check the gallbladder each year by ultrasound and have another course of bile acid treatment if stones come back.

Bile duct stones

A stone in the bile duct is like the Queen of Spades in the card game Black Maria: you get rid of it at all costs.

If a stone is found when the gallbladder is being removed it can be removed at that time. If the stone is found after the operation the surgeon may leave the T-tube drain in place. After about six weeks the track of the T-tube is used to steer a basket up to the stone, which can be ensnared and pulled out through the skin.

Dissolving stones

Another way of removing a stone in the bile duct soon after surgery is to inject a liquid, which dissolves cholesterol, through the T-tube. After a few days many of the smaller stones at the bottom of the bile duct are dissolved away or made smaller so that they pass on their own. The usual treatment is to inject a drug called mono-octanoin, but other drugs are being tested as well.

Half of the stones 7 mm (¼") or less across can be dissolved by this method and sometimes larger stones as well.

Catching stones in a basket

Another way is to attack the problem from the other end. You swallow an instrument called a flexible fibreoptic endoscope. The end is passed into the duodenum (small intestine) and through the instrument a wire is passed which can be made "electrically" live to cut or widen the entrance to the bile duct.

Stones in the bile duct can then be taken out by catching them in a wire basket or passing a tube with a balloon on the end of it up the bile ducts, blowing it up above the stone, and then dragging it down. Sometimes just making the cut in the entrance makes it wide enough for stones to pass out on their own.

Can't take an anaesthetic?

In people who cannot have a general anaesthetic, bile duct stones may be removed by the endoscope, even when the gallbladder is still in place with stones in it. If stones cannot be removed completely at the time it is possible to place a fine plastic tube in the bile duct with the end above the stone and bring the other end out through the duodenum, stomach, gullet, and nose. A drug, mono-octanoin, can be carefully injected to dissolve away stones. Another treatment is to take bile acids by mouth. This will eventually dissolve about half the non-chalky common bile duct stones, but it does take a long time.

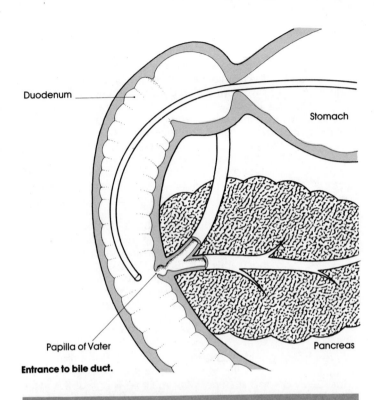

Duodenum

Stomach

Papilla of Vater

Pancreas

Entrance to bile duct.

Smashing ideas for the future

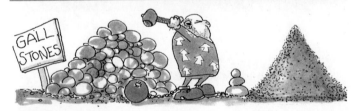

Crushing stones

As old-style convicts knew, stones can be broken down to very fine gravel and dust if they are bashed long enough.

A strong wire basket in which stones are caught has been designed which can be tightened to crush the stones to fragments. It is a difficult technique and tends to frighten the doctors using it!

Sound waves

In the same way that an opera singer's voice can shatter a glass, sound waves can be focused to cause similar damage. This was found by the Dornier aircraft company when machinery inside their planes was damaged by shockwaves even though the fuselage was intact.

These German engineers developed a system that formed controlled shockwaves and then focused them by a reflector to that they could smash stones inside patients. The first systems involved sending the soundwaves through water baths, and was so painful that an anaesthetic was needed. They were best for stones in the kidneys or urinary tract. Later different systems were used, sending shockwaves through air, and these are more suitable for gallstones.

This is a very new technique. In 1987 a doctor in Munich reported good success with 200 patients. After a few thousand shocks over about 45 minutes stones were reduced to a very small size, and the debris left in the gallbladder was then treated by taking bile acids by mouth. The same procedure may be useful for bile duct stones. First the stones need to be located, usually by ultrasound for the gallbladder.

Lasers

An even more recent idea is to use lasers. The laser fibre tip is brought up close to the stone, and direct contact can be made using a sapphire end. After multiple firings of the laser over about five minutes stones can be pulverised, but the procedure does mean getting close to the stone and holding it still, which may be a big problem.

Ether treatment makes a comeback

There are a lot of very powerful solvents that will make cholesterol dissolve, but we don't use most of them in people because they are so poisonous. Impatient doctors have never liked to have to wait months or years to see if bile acids will dissolve stones.

At the Mayo Clinic in the USA they tried sticking a needle through the skin into the gallbladder and injecting ether. A good success was achieved in dissolving stones. The hazards are that ethers are explosive anaesthetics, and can make the patient sleepy and something of a fire hazard if anyone smokes nearby!

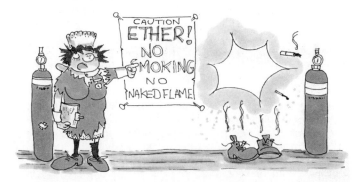

What about gallbladder cancer?

Gallbladder cancer is not very common. This is fortunate because it is a very difficult problem for doctors to treat successfully. About nine out of 10 cancers happen in gallbladders which contain stones and also do not contract properly. The only sort of cancers that can definitely be cured — by removing the gallbladder — are those which are so small and found so early that they can only be detected by the pathologist with a microscope, which means that the gallbladder was taken out for another reason.

This is such a depressing condition for surgeons that it has been suggested it should be prevented by removing all gallbladders with stones in them! This would, of course, be impossible because it would mean testing everyone again and again. People without symptoms would be asked to have operations they didn't want. In any case there would not be enough surgeons to do all the operations as well as all the other operations that have to be carried out.

It has been worked out that if all the gallbladders with stones were removed in a country like Britain there would be more deaths from the operation than lives saved by cancer prevention. It is different with the American Red Indians, who seem to have a much higher rate of gallbladder cancer so that energetic treatment of all their gallstones may be more useful.

10 Alcohol and liver disease

Drinking habits in different countries

How much you drink and what effect it has on your liver are important but often misunderstood topics. We know that the quantity of alcohol drunk in a country is directly related to the amount of liver disease. It does not matter whether the preferred national tipple is beer, wine, or spirits, the important thing is how much alcohol is drunk. Though you can damage your liver from drinking alcohol, it is not usually cirrhosis that develops but other types of inflammation, and these will clear up if you stop drinking completely.

Do we drink too much in Britain?

There has been a lot of publicity recently about people in Britain drinking more alcohol and the problems that go along with it. The change has probably had many causes but the main one must have been taxation policies which have made alcohol relatively much cheaper as its total price has not kept up with inflation. People in Britain have drunk rather less beer on licensed premises and much more wine at home and in restaurants in recent years, which confuses the issue as brewers closed pubs because of lack of trade at a time of increasing alcohol intake.

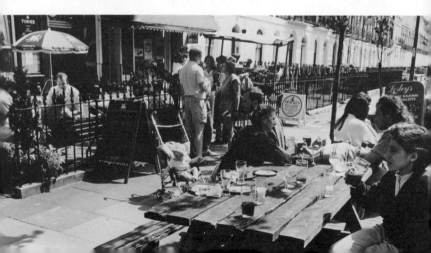

Our ancestors were pretty heavy drinkers

The picture is not all gloom. Britain is well down the world league for alcoholic liver disease, and France, Italy, and Germany have much worse problems. The much trumpetted rise in alcohol consumption happened after 1950, but this period of post-war austerity was a time at which alcohol intake in Britain was the lowest ever recorded.

Taxation records accurately show how much alcohol was officially consumed over the last three centuries in England and Wales. The total amount drunk can be divided by the known population at different times to give an average intake per head, which was enormously high in the 19th century and even higher still in the 18th century.

There was a continuous fall in alcohol intake since records began at the end of the 17th century until 1950, mainly explained by increasing price. Cheap gin was the chemical holiday from the wretched conditions of the city poor in the past, and it seems clear that most people were drunk most of the time between the restoration of Charles II and the Victorian age. It seemed unlikely that sobriety was particularly common before Cromwell either! Figures for the 1980s suggest that alcohol consumption may have levelled off again.

Safe limits

Alcohol intake is calculated in units. A half pint of beer, a glass of wine, or a single measure of spirits all contain one unit. For adults the average British intake is approximately 20 units a week (10 pints for a beer drinker).

To avoid any physical harm a healthy man shouldn't drink more than 21 units a week and a healthy woman more than 14 units a week. These are official recommendations. There is some evidence that at these levels physical health is actually improved, and the moderate drinker may expect to live a little longer than the teetotaller.

If you drink more than the "safe limit"

In practice liver problems do not usually occur until after a period of much heavier drinking than these limits. One definition of definite alcoholism which may be expected to

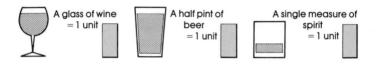

Average British intake (per week)		
20 units		

Safe limit		
Men		21 units per week
Women	14 units per week	

Safe drinking limits.

cause liver problems is a regular intake of eight units daily for 10 years or more.

It is, however, important to avoid very heavy drinking because this can cause acute and fatal liver disease even after short periods. Although liver damage is unpredictable it can be very severe. A survey of 600 patients with alcoholism living in Scotland identified one man who died of alcoholic cirrhosis at the age of 21.

For an individual with liver disease of any sort complete abstaining from alcohol is recommended to speed recovery. If the damage was caused by alcohol in the first place, lifelong avoidance of alcohol is the only safe advice. Though "low-alcohol" beverages may be useful to help replace intake of stronger drinks for normal people, they may be dangerous in alcoholic liver disease because the alcohol content may still be considerable. One brand of "low-alcohol" cider for instance has 3% alcohol, which is as much as some conventional beers!

A 33 year old man with moderate liver damage was an alcoholic who agreed to be treated to help him dry out. This included taking tablets of disulfiram (Antabuse). Taking these tablets strengthens the resolve not to drink because if alcohol is taken poisons build up in the body and make the patient feel terrible. He gave up his heavy drinking of ordinary beer, but his social life was the pub and he found he could drink one brand of low-alcohol beer without problems. This was certified to contain less than 0.1% alcohol. People being the adventurous experimenters they are, he then tried another brand with 0.9% alcohol. This quickly caused abdominal pain, vomiting, and general collapse of stout party. His physician advised him again to stick to soft drinks at the next consultation.

How alcohol affects the liver

Alcohol is a simple compound with the chemical formula C_2H_5OH. It is broken down by enzymes in the liver to water and carbon dioxide. If your liver is damaged the system does not work so well and alcohol levels in the blood — which cause the mental effects which are the reason for drinking — remain high for longer. This explains why alcoholics who have cirrhosis may actually drink less alcohol because they become drunk more quickly.

How your liver adapts

If you drink alcohol regularly the first effect on the liver is that it increases in size. Also, the various liver enzymes, which break chemicals down, including those enzymes that break down alcohol, have to speed up their action. This means that if you are taking medicine for something, it may not work well because the drugs, like alcohol, are broken down more rapidly and may go by different routes. One enzyme which is affected by alcohol is called gamma-glutamyl transferase and higher than normal levels of this are commonly found in the blood of heavy drinkers.

How your liver is damaged

Actual changes to the liver takes a variety of shapes. *Fat* is laid down in the cells, interfering with their function. *Inflammation*, causing some liver cells to die and the accumulation of many white blood cells and abnormal proteins, may be so severe that it is termed *alcoholic hepatitis*. *Excess iron* may be laid down in the liver. These changes should all disappear if you survive to stop drinking alcohol.

Cirrhosis

The next stage is the development of *cirrhosis*. This is permanent liver damage with some liver cells dying off, others regrowing, and heavy fibrous scar tissue laid down in bands to form nodules. This is not the end of the story. Cirrhosis may not cause many problems, or it may progress to liver failure with jaundice, coma, and death. Finally, alcoholic cirrhosis may transform into a liver cancer or *hepatoma*, for which you have little chance of being treated effectively.

How the doctor knows you are a heavy drinker

The doctor's often impossible goal is to detect alcohol abuse early enough to prevent your developing any permanent physical harm.

A doctor would suspect alcohol abuse when patients have unexplained frequent falls and fractures, a poor work record, and early morning nausea and retching. Almost any complaint may be caused by alcohol abuse, and people are frequently vague and deceitful about their habits.

A 45 year old woman was admitted to hospital because of numerous complaints. She wanted to have an amenity bed in a side-ward, and as is often the case with patients with drinking problems, she converted this into a little "home from home". It was noted on a ward round that she had brought in a supply of soft drinks, not at all unusual for a patient. However, she had a whole litre jug of tomato juice. An astute young doctor invited himself to sample this and confirmed his suspicion that this was indeed a Bloody Mary, with a very high vodka content.

Telltale signs

Unkempt appearance, heavy cigarette use, and erratic behaviour may indicate to the doctor that someone drinks heavily. People who smell of alcohol in the morning before pub opening time are regarded as alcoholics until proved otherwise. And their blood can be checked for a high alcohol level.

A 53 year old woman smelled of alcohol in a morning clinic. When asked about this she explained that a small amount of lager had been left over from a can opened the previous evening and she had tidied it up. Her blood alcohol level was 80 mg/dl (over the limit for driving). She had either been drinking very heavily indeed the previous night, or more likely she had drunk a couple of pints that morning.

Tests

The doctor may send you for routine "liver function" tests, which may show changes in your liver. A blood count will often show that the red blood cells are larger than they should be because alcohol can interfere with blood formation by the bone marrow.

To prove the exact nature of the damage to your liver, and to predict the outcome, a liver biopsy will be carried out. This is done by inserting a needle into the liver and removing a little liver tissue, which is then examined. If for some reason a liver biopsy cannot be done, a test called an isotope liver scan is performed to see whether you have cirrhosis and to look at the blood flow through the liver.

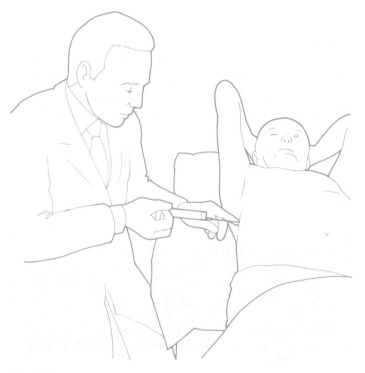

Liver biopsy.

Can alcoholism be treated?

The first treatment for alcoholism is to stop drinking alcohol. Going into hospital is the best thing, because generally people have no trouble giving up alcohol in the surroundings of a hospital ward. Tests, such as liver biopsy, can be done, and medical and social problems can be dealt with.

Withdrawal effects from alcohol are sometimes troublesome, and may make a person anxious and tremulous. Taking anti-anxiety or tranquillising drugs in the form of tablets, like propranolol or chlormethiazole (Hemineverin), is helpful for a short time. Alcoholic patients should not be given tranquillisers to take home because they may start to drink again and the combination of drink and drugs can be lethal. This combination was responsible for the British rock group The Who becoming a trio instead of a foursome.

Delirium tremens

Sometimes withdrawal effects are very bad, and cause hallucinations and fits. This is *delirium tremens* (DTs) and needs to be treated quickly with drugs by injection. Most commonly used are shots of diazepam, and chlormethiazole by drip for a day or two. Some of the problems of the alcoholic are caused by poor nourishment and high doses of vitamins B and C by injection are needed.

Disulfiram tablets

To strengthen the resolve of the reformed drinker treatment with disulfiram tablets is often used. This means taking a tablet in the morning, when most people feel least like a drink, but it acts all day long to cover the evening when temptation is strongest. The drug blocks one of the liver enzymes and so alcohol is only partly broken down. A chemical called acetaldehyde builds up in the blood to levels which are poisonous and makes the person very unwell. This treatment can kill if alcohol is drunk, and it concentrates the alcoholic's mind wonderfully to be told this.

The best results long term come only if the alcoholic decides to reform, but medical and social support are also needed to get good results. Voluntary contact with Alcoholics Anonymous is very useful.

Cirrhosis

When a person has cirrhosis fluid may cause the body to swell. This is treated by restricting the amount of salt in the diet and by taking diuretic tablets. If the abdomen is severely swollen a plastic tube can be inserted through the skin to drain off fluid continuously. Treatment is also started to stop this fluid returning.

Mental changes can be improved by avoiding drugs which affect brain action and by reducing the amount of protein in the diet, as it is protein breakdown products which cause part of the problem. Certain drugs may help to reduce confusion too.

Internal Bleeding

One of the most difficult conditions to deal with when a person has cirrhosis is internal bleeding, which may be from ulcers or from enlarged veins at the bottom of the gullet. A temporary solution is to give a blood transfusion, together with treatment with vitamin K and fresh blood plasma, which will help blood clot better. The stomach is examined inside by fibreoptic endoscope as soon as possible to find the cause of bleeding.

If there are veins at the bottom of the gullet these can be injected at the time to block them off – alcohol itself can be used, by a nice paradox! If bleeding continues then a balloon at the end of a tube can be left blown up in the gullet for a day or so to flatten the veins, and further treatment given to reduce pressure in the veins. If this is not the answer then an operation to cut all the guilty veins or to divert the blood flow is the last resort. This is a desperate measure for a dangerous disease.

Sometimes internal bleeding comes from an ordinary peptic ulcer. This is easily healed by taking tablets, provided the patient survives the bleed.

People with cirrhosis may have health problems which do not improve with treatment or rapidly worsen. This may just be the disease getting worse, but cancer may have developed. Though the tests are limited, liver biopsy or scanning can help. Even simpler, many liver cancers (hepatomas) make large amounts of an abnormal protein called *alpha-fetoprotein*, which can easily be found in your blood. For someone who has alcoholic cirrhosis with hepatoma, no curative treatment is available, but help can and will be given to control symptoms.

Alcoholics with cirrhosis sometimes object that since the liver damage will not go away they might as well go on drinking. This is wrong. Continuing to drink alcohol causes even more illness and shortens life in this condition. The alcohol intake in

> **Problems worsen each other:** A man in his 60s with alcoholic cirrhosis was admitted to hospital for treatment of fluid. But did not make good progress and became more confused and lethargic. It was noticed that he was becoming increasingly anaemic for no clear reason and an endoscopy was performed. He had a bleeding duodenal ulcer and the blood from this had effectively turned his intestine into a human black pudding. The protein breakdown for this had affected his brain. When he was treated for the ulcer, and with a low protein diet and lactulose to reduce protein breakdown he became alert and grateful.

France fell dramatically after the occupation in 1940 because of the effect of the country being full of Nazis. It rose to celebratory levels after the liberation in 1944. During the war years, deaths from alcoholic cirrhosis fell sharply, but reached their former level again after the war. The logical conclusion is that the Frenchmen with cirrhosis who stopped or reduced their alcohol intake survived longer — and that message should be heeded on this side of the Channel.

11 Viruses and liver disease

Viruses are the smallest of the infectious germs which cause disease. They are very simple and are very difficult to kill or even to treat with drugs. Much effort to stop the damage caused by harmful viruses is directed to immunising people against them. Immunisation is very effective in controlling some virus diseases, such as polio and measles, and was largely the reason that smallpox was stamped out in the 1970s.

Most of the viruses which damage your liver are spread directly from person to person, but sometimes animals can infect people.

Hepatitis A
- **Very common**
- **Usually mild in children**
- **Worse in adults**
- **Appetite goes**
- **You feel awful**
- **Jaundice comes and goes**
- **You recover completely**

Hepatitis A

Hepatitis A is called infectious hepatitis, and it is a very common disease. It is seen less often in wealthy countries than in developing countries and thrives where the climate is warm and sanitation is poor.

How you get it

It is spread by poor hygiene. The viruses pass out with the faeces and can contaminate the hands and so be passed on to others through contamination of food. Outbreaks occur in schools. If you have been infected and recovered from hepatitis A you will have lifelong immunity, so that you can never again catch the disease.

When does it show up?

The virus does not show at once but takes at least a week before it causes problems. Sometimes the infection does not show itself for six weeks. In children the illness is often mild and makes them feel off colour, with some diarrhoea and vomiting. Often jaundice occurs (but not always) and occasionally the child develops a rash. It is easy to diagnose when epidemics occur. If there is any doubt about whether you have it a blood test will give the answer.

What happens?

In adults the disease is much worse. First you lose your appetite, and smokers are generally revolted by tobacco smoke. Then you feel awful and lose stamina. But the good news is that after some weeks in which jaundice comes and then goes, you recover to perfect health.

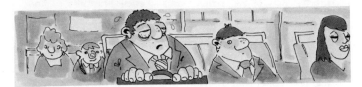

How is it treated?

There is no particular treatment to make the illness go away quickly, but you are told to avoid alcohol for some months so your fragile liver isn't damaged further. Jaundice and skin itching are sometimes a nuisance and treatment with cortisone controls this.

In about one in a hundred adults with hepatitis the liver is severely damaged and there is liver failure. This means you need intensive hospital care to stay alive. Even then when you get better your recovery is complete.

Protection from the virus

If people who have not had hepatitis A themselves in the past are going to come in contact with the virus, they can have an injection of *hyperimmune globulin*. This gives them short term protection. It is made from the blood of patients who have recently recovered from hepatitis A, and helps stop the virus gaining hold. About half the middle aged and older people of Britain have been exposed to hepatitis A at some time in their younger life and have immunity — won't get it. Children and young adults have less protection because the disease is becoming less frequent.

A four-year-old at nursery school became generally difficult one summer. She was irritable and had diarrhoea for a short time. A nettle rash came and went, and the doctor thought that the problem was allergy to strawberries and "end-of-termitis". She recovered and went to Belgium with her family. Her mother — a secondary school teacher — also felt very run down but thought this was not surprising in view of the tiring effect of a poorly child and working full time at the end of the school year. Mum did not enjoy her holiday sightseeing at all. After a few days Dad noticed that not only had she got a remarkably good "suntan" for northern Europe but that her eyes had gone yellow! When the family went home they discovered that there had been an outbreak of infectious hepatitis A at the nursery school and their daughter had obviously brought this home. Father was not at risk because he was immune after having hepatitis A in childhood. He also could clearly remember his family being fed up with him until the reason for his fractious behaviour was diagnosed!

How you feel

Anyone who has viral hepatitis is likely to feel very tired and depressed. But the doctor will reassure you that these feelings will all get better eventually. No special diet helps though you often have a very poor appetite and lose weight because of not eating much. It is very important to keep drinking fluids so you don't become dehydrated. In the old days bed rest used to be recommended. But there is no advantage in staying in bed if you feel like getting up and pottering about. You are the best one to decide what you will eat and whether you need to rest.

Hepatitis B
- **More harmful than hepatitis A**
- **Spread through blood and sexual intercourse**
- **People at risk are drug addicts, prostitutes, and homosexuals**

Hepatitis B

Hepatitis B is caused by a much more damaging virus than hepatitis A. But this is mercifully less common in Britain and is becoming even less so. Hepatitis B is a very important problem for the whole world. Though only about one out of every 1000 people in the UK and USA has been in contact with the virus, in some Eastern countries like Taiwan as many as one out of every seven people is in contact with it.

How do you get it?

The virus is spread by human blood and by sexual intercourse, and occasionally by saliva. It can also be spread from mothers to their newborn children especially in Chinese people. Because blood and blood products can spread the disease all transfusion blood is tested for hepatitis B virus before it is used. Spread of the virus this way is not a problem in Britain now.

Who is at risk?

Drug addicts are not so careful with themselves, and when they share syringes and needles they easily spread hepatitis B. Any sort of sexual intercourse with men can spread the virus. Prostitutes and homosexuals are especially as risk because they usually have a large number of partners, and they are very likely to have an infected partner.

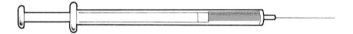

Infection

Infection with hepatitis B virus can have several results. Some people may have no illness at all. The virus clears out of their system completely, and they become immune. Others may never be ill but become carriers, and they can infect others. There is a test for this.

Sometimes the virus causes an illness that lasts a short time, similar to hepatitis A. In 1986 this happened to 1300 Britons and 30 died. There were 800 cases in 1987. It takes between six weeks and six months after infection for the liver to become inflamed. Sometimes this inflammation persists and eventually causes cirrhosis.

Cancer

The most serious of all the problems caused by the hepatitis B virus is liver cancer. Although this killing disease is not a big problem in the United Kingdom, it is thought to be the commonest cancer in men in the world.

Protection against the virus

Hepatitis B can be prevented by people being immunised against it. Three injections spread over six months will give you almost complete protection. Immunisation is given to people at risk, such as medical staff who care for infected patients and handle their blood. Someday it may be possible to immunise the whole world to wipe out the virus altogether.

Another infection

A person infected by hepatitis B virus may also catch another viral illness called *delta hepatitis*. This germ is one cause of long term liver inflammation after infection with hepatitis B.

How does it spread?

How hepatitis B virus spreads can be a puzzle because of the long time it takes to show up.

Sheila lived alone in a village in the north east of England. She developed acute hepatitis B, but she recovered completely. Her neighbour Wanda, who was a close friend, developed the same problem a few weeks later. They both denied using any illegal drugs, had had no injections in the previous year, and said they did not have a common sexual partner. Wanda's husband suggested that sharing sewing needles might have spread the infection. But this did not explain how Sheila had contracted the illness in the first place. He himself had no illness and tests were negative in him. It then emerged that Sheila was separated from her husband, who was a heroin addict living in London. He had visited her four months before she became ill to attempt a reconciliation. Both women said again that they did not use any illegal drugs, and Wanda said she hadn't had any sexual contact with Sheila's husband. Eighteen months later Wanda was convicted of sending cannabis by post to her own husband who was a seaman. This suggested that what she had said before may not have been the whole truth, and that one way or another Sheila's husband had indeed given the infection to both women.

Hepatitis non-A non-B

The dustbin term, hepatitis non-A non-B, describes a third group of viruses which can cause hepatitis and be spread in different ways. One way is by blood transfusion. This cannot be prevented fully because there is no test to screen blood from donors properly. Possibly because our volunteer donor system in Britain is different from that in the United States, we do not have the problem that they do in North America, where non-A non-B hepatitis quite often develops after a blood transfusion.

What happens?

This usually shows up as a mild, short attack of hepatitis some weeks or months after a blood transfusion. Sometimes there is also persisting inflammation of the liver.

Other viruses

Yellow fever

Yellow fever is a serious viral illness, spread by mosquito bites, which is common in the tropics. Anyone who goes to areas where it is common should be immunised before going.

Viruses caught from animals

There are some very sinister hepatitis viruses which can spread from animals to humans. For example, an epidemic of *Ebola fever* in Zaire was probably started when soldiers fighting jungle wars were in contact with monkeys or apes. This outbreak quickly killed more than 180 of the 200 people infected. Monkeys used in research caused deaths in laboratory workers in Germany, from a form of viral hepatitis called *Marburg disease*.

Glandular fever

Glandular fever is usually easy to spot because the symptoms are a sore throat, fever, severe lethargy, and enlarged lymph nodes and spleen. Sometimes it affects the body in a different way so that the liver is the main target. If your doctor suspects this, it can be proved by tests and by finding unusual white cells in the blood. Other viruses causing general illnesses such as measles may sometimes also attack the liver in the same way.

Other problems

Infants can have jaundice

Infants may have jaundice after birth, particularly if they are premature, but they should get over it completely. In some infants jaundice does not go away. There are two reasons. The infant may have *neonatal hepatitis*, probably caused by a virus, or the bile ducts may be damaged or not formed properly. Surgery, including having a liver transplant, may be used for the child to survive if the problem is serious.

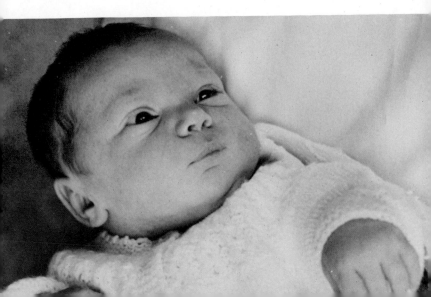

Blood infection

When your blood is infected with bacteria the liver can filter the bacteria out to help you to recover. But sometimes the germs thrive in the liver itself. When that happens pus collects in the liver and you develop a *liver abscess*. You can take powerful antibiotics, and the pus can be drained out by needle or operation. But these treatments are not always successful.

Weil's disease

Weil's disease is the result of being infected with bacteria found in the urine of rats and dogs. This is an occupational risk for farmers, sewer workers, and dockers. It causes jaundice and a form of meningitis, but once the cause is recognised treatment is usually effective.

12 Auto-immune liver disease

After alcohol and viruses, auto-immunity is the commonest cause of long term liver disease. This means that your body reacts against itself and the liver is damaged. Why this happens is a mystery, but illness of this type is much commoner in women than men and can be linked with other diseases such as colitis. Primary biliary cirrhosis and chronic active hepatitis are the main types of auto-immune disease.

Primary biliary cirrhosis

In primary biliary cirrhosis the small bile ducts in the liver are inflamed and damaged. Eventually, in severe cases, they disappear and cause cirrhosis. Because bile does not flow out of the liver normally various consequences follow. Your skin itches, and this can be so bad that it keeps you awake. You might have diarrhoea and get thinner because your body cannot absorb fat properly.

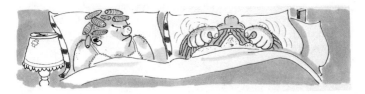

In primary biliary cirrhosis, certain vitamins which are absorbed with fats are also not taken up. This can cause bone disease (vitamin D), night blindness (vitamin A), and bleeding disorders (vitamin K). The skin darkens, jaundice eventually develops, and cholesterol (the fatty substance in cells) is laid down in yellow plaques in the skin. Almost everyone who has biliary cirrhosis has a particular substance called *mitochondrial antibody*, in the blood, and this provides one test for the disease. Even early in the disease, a liver biopsy — a sample of liver removed by a needle and examined under a microscope — will be abnormal.

How is it treated?

Many cases are mild and need no special treatment. For some people, replacing the vitamin deficiencies is the answer. If itching is a problem you can take antihistamine tablets like terfenadine, or cholestyramine which binds with bile acids, or have ultraviolet light treatment. If the disease is very severe you might have to consider a liver transplant.

Many different "curative" or disease-controlling treatments have been tested, but none has been so effective and safe that all doctors believe in it. There are several drugs being investigated: prednisolone, which must be used with great care because of the chance of making bone disease worse; the powerful immunosuppressive drug cyclosporin; and ursode-oxycholic acid, more familiar as a treatment for gallstones.

Chronic active hepatitis

Chronic active hepatitis is a different type of inflammation which damages liver cells. But it can also eventually lead to cirrhosis. Sometimes it starts out as an illness like hepatitis before it becomes persistent, so virus causes have to be ruled out. Damage to the liver caused by drinking too much alcohol can cause a similar illness.

Tests

Blood tests usually show that the blood has persistently high levels of an enzyme called transaminase. Most people who have chronic active hepatitis also have particular *antibodies* in the blood. You might have a liver biopsy to prove you have this disease.

How is it treated?

The usual treatment is with the drug prednisolone perhaps together with an immunosuppressive drug, azathioprine. But side effects are difficult to deal with because high doses of drugs are needed to damp down the disease.

13 Poisons, drugs and herbs

Sometimes people accidentally or deliberately take large doses of chemicals which damage the liver.

Carbon tetrachloride

Carbon tetrachloride, a useful dry cleaning fluid, can kill liver cells when drunk or inhaled in large quantities. This is notorious but not common.

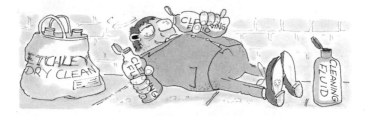

Paracetamol

Much more common is *paracetamol* overdose. This painkiller is rightly freely available, because when it is used correctly it does what it is supposed to do and is safe. But when you take too much paracetamol it is very dangerous indeed. The liver is swamped by paracetamol and it cannot cope.

A poisonous byproduct is made in the liver which kills liver cells. This is even more deadly for heavy drinkers. If you can get to hospital within 12 hours the amount of paracetamol in your blood can be tested. If it is dangerously high an antidote can be given. After 12 hours the harm will have been done to your liver.

Liver damage can also be caused by medical treatment.

A 21 year old man had a row with his girlfriend and took a whole bottle of paracetamol tablets. He later became anxious, reported the event, and was admitted to hospital 18 hours after he had taken the tablets. He was apparently well and while in hospital made it up with his girl. Forty eight hours after he had taken the tablets he began to feel dizzy and sick. He developed liver failure and then went into a coma. He died a week later, despite the doctors and nurses doing everything they could for him. His truly was an accidental death — he had never really intended to die but only to "teach someone a lesson".

Anaesthesia

Halothane, an anaesthetic used in surgery, causes liver inflammation if used often.

Tranquillisers

Some tranquillisers like *chlorpromazine* may cause a type of hepatitis. They may also interfere with bile flow and cause jaundice and itching.

Sex hormones

Sex hormones may cause jaundice. That is why the lowest possible amounts are used in the "pill" and in hormone replacement therapy. And why it is just plain crazy for athletes to take high doses of male hormones.

Herbs

Though herbal remedies are thought to be safe if not so powerful as usual medicine, this is sometimes untrue. For instance, the herbal concoction known as bush tea causes severe liver disease by making blood clots form in the veins of the liver. This is not just a problem in South America and India, because similar infusions are commonly drunk on the mainland of Europe and to a lesser extent in Britain.

A teenage boy came down with severe ulcerative colitis. This is inflammation of the bowel and can be treated by medical drugs. His parents objected to drugs and stopped them. Instead they gave him many cups of *comfrey tea*. Then he got worse and went back to the doctor. Unfortunately, his liver was so badly damaged by this herbal "remedy" that he had cirrhosis.

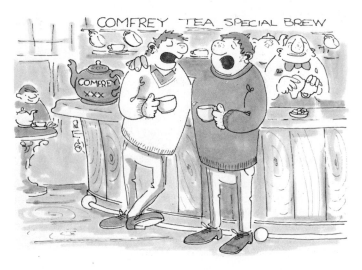

14 Treatment of liver failure

When you have chronic liver failure there is bleeding, too much fluid, and mental confusion, and these have to be treated. If the liver failure gets worse, more treatment is needed. The same is true of short term liver damage caused by viral hepatitis and paracetamol overdose.

What can be done?

You are given intensive treatment and fed through a drip to help you to survive. Sometimes doctors try to purify the blood. Part of the blood is taken out of your body and passed through charcoal or resin particles. These absorb poison before the blood is returned to your body.

Transplants

When liver damage is so bad as to be life-threatening, the liver can be replaced by transplantation. For this, you need a suitable donor. And so that the body doesn't reject the new liver, you have to take immunosuppresive drugs for the rest of your life.

The results of transplantation are pretty good. Though 20% to 30% of people who receive liver transplants die in the first year after operation (often because they are very ill before the transplant), the remainder can expect to live useful lives. The results of transplantation are better when it is carried out in children.

15 Liver cancer

Liver cancer, or hepatoma, often occurs in people who also have cirrhosis because of alcoholism, or infection with the hepatitis B virus, or too much iron in the liver (haemochromatosis). When someone with cirrhosis gets worse for some unexplained reason, the doctor will consider cancer. The blood can be tested for the amount of *alpha-feto protein* and a liver biopsy done.

How is it treated?

Drug treatment doesn't always work, but new drugs are being developed. A liver transplant may be considered if the cancer hasn't spread outside the liver. If a person with hepatoma doesn't have cirrhosis, then the part of the liver in which the tumour lies can be removed and the results are usually good. Before the operation a CT scanning test would be done to make sure there would be enough normal liver left.

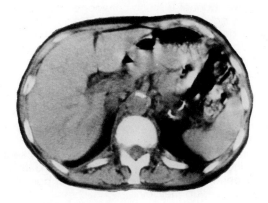

Scan showing a cross section through the body. This shows a normal liver.

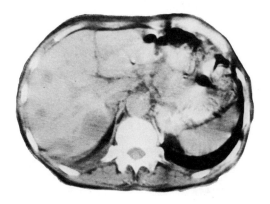

Scan shows several patches of a different colour due to cancer.

Secondary liver cancer

Secondary liver cancer is much commoner in Britain. Because there is a very good blood supply to the liver, cancer cells from the intestine and other parts of the body often reach the liver and grow there. This is especially true when there are growths in the large bowel (rectum and colon), stomach, and pancreas. Doctors can detect this type of spread in various ways: by checking the blood levels of certain enzymes or by checking for a blood protein which indicates that cancer has spread. The liver can be examined by ultrasound, or an isotope scan, or CT scanning. A liver biopsy can usually show what type of cancer it is.

It is very important to know whether there are any secondary cancers in the liver before any surgery is considered for the primary cancer. This type of spreading cancer can sometimes be controlled by drug therapy.

16 Tests for liver disease

If you have liver disease the symptoms which you describe to your doctor provide the clues. These symptoms may not be caused by liver disease, however, but by some other problem. To make sure that you have liver disease you will be examined for *physical signs* and various tests or *investigations* will be done.

Physical signs

Jaundice — yellowish skin — is often obvious, but a whole host of other skin problems may show up in a person whose liver stops doing its job properly.

- Your skin may become thin and papery.
- You bruise easily.
- Clusters of small blood vessels show up on your face and trunk.
- Your nails can change too, going white and perhaps becoming very curved.
- Your ankles and belly may swell.
- Your ability to think and speak may become slow, and a poor memory causes you to contradict yourself.

When this problem with the brain is severe people have tremors and drift into coma.

In men hormone changes can cause problems. You may lose your sex drive, the testicles shrink, your beard grows slower, and you may grow breasts.

Cholesterol can build up in the skin to form yellowish lumps. Sometimes the liver enlarges and becomes hard so that the doctor can easily feel it in the upper right side of your abdomen. But usually the liver is of normal size or even small.

Rarely, but even more important, the spleen gets larger and can be felt in the upper left side of the abdomen.

> **Signs of liver disease**
> - **Yellow skin (jaundice)**
> - **Thin, papery skin**
> - **Bruising**
> - **Blood vessels on face and trunk**
> - **White, curved nails**
> - **Swollen ankles and belly**
> - **Slow thinking and speaking**
> - **Poor memory**

Blood tests

Your doctor can discover a lot of useful information about your health by examining a sample of blood in a laboratory. But unfortunately even severe, often fatal, liver disease does not necessarily show in this way. Cirrhosis may not show up on the so-called "liver function" tests at all.

Bilirubin

Bilirubin — the yellowness of the blood serum — is commonly high in the blood in liver disease and repeated tests are often made to assess whether the liver is showing signs of recovery.

Enzymes

When the liver is damaged it produces more quantities of some enzymes, and these spill over into the blood so the blood has more than normal. These include transaminases and alkaline phosphatase, and you may be told that you have high levels of one or both categories. Again repeated tests will show how quickly your liver is returning to normal.

Albumin

Albumin, which is a useful protein, is made in the liver and the amount in the blood falls if the liver stops working for any reason.

Globulin

Your body defends itself from attack in different ways. Lymphocytes, which are the white cells of the blood produced in the lymph nodes and spleen, are very important. There are two main kinds of lymphocytes.

One sort is responsible for mopping up germs and cancer cells, and clusters of these can be seen in diseased tissue under the microscope.

The other sort of lymphocytes produces different proteins which help to stop inflammation. These proteins — immune globulins — coat undersireble cells and make them harmless and easy to destroy. Two types of the *immune globulins* that are specially important in liver disease are called *IgG* and *IgM*.

Cholesterol

The liver makes a lot of cholesterol. We all know that having a lot of cholesterol in the blood is generally linked with heart disease. But this is not usually the case in liver disease.

If your liver is not working properly cholesterol is not passed out into the bile, and it builds up in the body. The cholesterol circulates in the blood attached to an abnormal protein, and forms small lumps in the skin, but does not seem to do much harm to the arteries.

Urea

Urea is a harmless product which is made in the liver when protein is broken down. If the liver does not make urea properly, less urea is carried in the blood. Other toxic protein breakdown products accumulate instead, and these may affect the functioning of the brain.

Electrolytes

Electrolytes are salts. In liver disease levels of both *sodium* and *potassium* tend to be low in the blood, sometimes causing difficulties in their own right. For instance, not enough potassium affects the rhythm of your heart and very low sodium is linked to brain swelling.

Treatment

You can take potassium salts by mouth. Or you can take drugs to stop your body passing out potassium in the urine.

If you have low sodium it is very difficult to treat safely. Sometimes you will be given diuretic tablets.

Blood count

You can have *anaemia* because of bleeding or because your bone marrow isn't making enough red cells.

Viral infections

When infections damage the liver sometimes the germ responsible can be detected by laboratory tests. The best known example is the Australia antigen or *hepatitis B surface antigen*; its odd name is due to its having first been detected in an Australian aborigine.

There are also tests for antibodies which your body produces against particular liver infections, such as hepatitis A, hepatitis B, and glandular fever.

Occasionally virus particles can be found in blood, faeces, or in samples of the liver by using very powerful electron microscopes. But there is no proper test at all for what is mercifully a rare problem in Britain, the hepatitis non-A non-B, which can follow blood transfusion.

Other tests

Occasionally the liver is damaged because the body's chemistry is upset by iron or copper. There are blood tests for these metals.

It is easy to measure *alcohol* in the blood, breath, and urine.

Red herrings

Though the various blood tests can tell a lot about liver disease, the tests may show changes when other organs such as the heart or the bones are diseased. So sometimes repeated tests may be needed before your doctor can be certain about the exact cause of an illness.

17 Liver biopsy

One of the most reliable tests for suspected liver disease is liver biopsy.

The doctor can take samples of your liver by needle. These samples are examined with a microscope using special stains.

Before you have a biopsy the doctor will be sure certain conditions are met:

- There should be reasonable suspicion of liver disease.
- There should not be too much fluid in your abdomen, or the liver may just bounce off the end of the needle.
- Your blood should clot reasonably normally.

How it is done

Though a biopsy is done in hospital, you can usually go home afterwards. But some doctors like to keep you in overnight afterwards.

You lie flat on your back at the right edge of a bed and you place your right hand behind your head. To find where the liver lies the doctor bangs gently with his fingers to show dullness in the same way that the level of fluid in a barrel can be measured by tapping on the outside.

You have an injection of local anaesthetic to numb the skin. When this has taken effect, you hold your breath, a needle is quickly pushed into your liver, and suction is applied by a syringe.

Sometimes this is done two or three times to get a good sample. You then lie flat for about six hours and you are watched carefully to make sure there is no excess bleeding or leaking bile.

The biopsy sample is at once placed in a pot of evil-smelling formalin fixative and sent to the laboratory. Very thin slices are cut, the biopsy is stained to show the cells and fibres to best effect, and then it is examined carefully under a microscope shining electric light through the sample. It takes about two days for the laboratory to tell your doctor the results.

Cirrhosis, alcoholic liver disease, and cancer can be diagnosed by this very useful and safe method.

18 Why on earth did I go yellow?

If you are jaundiced, with yellow skin and eyeballs, by talking to you and examining you the doctor can usually find the cause. Sometimes, however, the cause may not be obvious. In these cases people are admitted to hospital because it is not at all clear what is wrong with them.

The possibilities

The two main possibilities are problems affecting the liver itself. Cirrhosis is one. Blocked bile ducts, which damage the liver by damming back the bile flow, is another.

These are called medical and surgical jaundice. If you have cirrhosis it is important not to operate since this does not cure the illness. But when the bile ducts are blocked whatever is obstructing them has to be removed quickly or the damage to your liver gets worse and you may die.

A 28 year old pregnant woman became jaundiced and itchy but didn't feel any pain in the later weeks of pregnancy. The doctor thought it was most likely that this was the common, harmless effect of hormone changes, and so no special tests were carried out until she had delivered a healthy baby. The jaundice did not improve. An ultrasound test showed that her bile ducts were mainly wide, but the lower end of the common bile duct was narrow. She was operated on and cancer was found in the pancreas. The pancreas was pressing on the common bile duct. An operation was carried out to protect the liver, but she died of cancer of the pancreas six months later. At least she had a little time with her new baby, and knew the outlook so she could help the family plan its life.

Surprises can happen the other way too. A 58 year old man was seen by a surgeon. The man had jaundice and fluid in his belly. He felt no pain, had not taken any drugs recently, and the doctor ruled out viral hepatitis. The man said that he drank little alcohol. He was admitted to hospital to drain the fluid and for tests. The doctor who checked him in noted that the man usually drank about three pints of beer when he went out, which did not seem important to this illness. The ultrasound test showed that the bile duct was normal, and another doctor was called in for advice. It was now discovered that the man spent every evening in the pub. He admitted that he drank five pints of beer every night — he was clearly an alcoholic. An isotope liver scan showed that he had almost certainly got cirrhosis. He got much better partly because of treatment for the fluid and a better diet — but largely because he kept out of licensed premises.

Tests

Liver ultrasound examination is the first test. This shows whether the bile ducts are wide because they are blocked. If they are, then you will probably have an operation. Other tests are necessary, too, so the surgeon knows what to expect when your belly is opened. If the bile ducts are not wide and do not become wide, then a liver biopsy is performed if it is safe to do so.

19 X rays and scans

X rays

X rays of your abdomen may show that your liver or spleen is enlarged. But they are often not very helpful.

CT scanning, in which a computer processes a set of *X* ray pictures taken at different angles, can give very good pictures of theliver. It can also show changes such as spreading cancer or increased sixze of the bile ducts.

It will also show large gallstones. In some special hospital units X rays of the blood supply are taken after injecting dye into the veins and arteries.

Isotope scans of the liver (see next page) showing radioactive particles in the liver being concentrated in the gall bladder after 15–20 minutes.

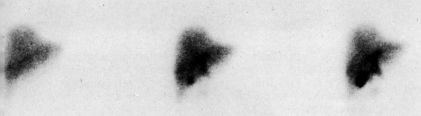

5 MIN   10 MIN   15 MIN

MEDICAL PHYSICS DEPARTMENT, DRYBURN HOSPITAL, DURHAM

20 MIN   25 MIN   30 MIN

Isotope scan

A way of showing up how the liver looks and works is to use tiny radioactive particles injected into a vein. These are taken up by liver cells lining the blood passages in the liver, whose job in life is mopping up unwanted substances in the blood.

A synthetic isotope called *technetium* is used. This is convenient and safe. The person lies under a gamma camera which detects the radiation and shows it as a picture. The normal liver shows up as a triangle with most of the liver on the right side. The spleen also takes up this isotope and appears like a large kidney bean on the left side.

If you have cirrhosis your liver is damaged and blood flow is abnormal. The isotope scan shows little of the isotope in the liver. But the spleen enlarges and takes up a lot more isotope. The isotope is not taken up by liver cancers so these show as gaps among the normal liver.

Ultrasound

Almost all *X* ray departments can now perform ultrasound. In ultrasound echo reflection is used instead of *X* ray penetration to outline the liver. These pictures are particularly helpful where a person has liver cancer, and large masses can be chosen for liver biopsy.

If bile flow is blocked the bile ducts increase in size. This is easily seen with liver ultrasound, though it may not be possible to prove the cause of the blockage, so that other tests will be needed to decide on the correct treatment.

20 Conclusion

Anyone who has read all the way through this book will have learned that diseases of the liver, gall bladder, and pancreas range from minor to life-threatening. An attack of viral hepatitis—infectious jaundice—may cause only a few days of inconvenience or it may plunge its victim into coma. Many people with gallstones are totally unaware they have them; others have repeated attacks of severe pain and sickness. So you sould not be surprised if your doctor is a bit cautious in forecasting the outcome when you first develop liver disease. He or she will probably want to arrange for some tests and wait for the results before answering your questions in detail.

Furthermore doctors quite often ask for tests to be done for liver disease in patients with rather vague symptoms. If this happens to you do not be alarmed; by asking for such tests your doctor is most likely to be trying to rule out liver disease. Fortunately the modern tests of liver function and the use of ultrasound and X-ray imaging have made it possible to test the liver very thoroughly. If your liver is given the all-clear then you can be pretty confident that the reassurance is correct.

Liver disease *is* complicated; but by learning more about it you are likely to be less worried by attendances at hospital. And we hope that this booklet will help you understand more clearly what your doctor has told you—and maybe suggest what questions to ask him.

Index

abscess, liver, 16, 76
age as gallstone risk, 36
albumin, 11, 87
alcohol, 15, 25
    as cause of disease, 26, 41
    and liver disease, 58–67
    safe limits of, 59–60
    see also alcoholism
Alcoholics Anonymous, 65
alcoholism, 23, 26, 60, 67, 79
    see also alcohol
anaemia, 20, 23, 39, 88
anaesthesia, 16, 80
auto-immune liver disease, 16,
    77–8

bile, 7, 9, 11, 14, 20, 21, 31, 77
    acids, 11, 13, 23, 28–9, 52–3, 55
    composition of, 30
    production of, 28–9
    see also bile ducts
bile ducts, 7, 9, 10
    blocked, 21, 23, 91
    removal of stones, 25, 48–9, 50,
        54–5
    stones in, 21, 25, 27, 28, 46
    see also bile
biliary colic, 27, 40
bilirubin, 14, 19, 20–1, 31, 32–3, 86
    conjugated, 14, 20, 21, 30
biopsy, liver, 64, 65, 77, 84, 90, 92
bleeding, 22–3, 82
    internal, 23, 66
blood
    cholesterol in, 13
    clotting, 11, 22, 23, 66, 81
    components of, 14
    infection, 76
    purification of, 82
    supply, 9, 11, 21
    tests, 44, 69, 78, 86
    transfusions, 66, 71, 74, 89
    see also anaemia; bleeding;
        bruising
bruising, 23, 85

calcium salts, 30, 31, 32
cancer
    of bile ducts, 28
    of gallbladder, 27, 57
    of liver, 16, 52, 62, 66, 72, 83, 90
    of pancreas, 21, 26
    secondary liver, 84
carbon tetrachloride, 79
causes
    of gallstones, 34–41
    of hepatitis, 69, 71–2, 74
    of jaundice, 19–21
    of liver damage, 15–16, 19–21
    of pancreatitis, 25–6
cholecystectomy, 48–51
cholecystitis, acute, 27, 41, 43, 46
cholesterol, 11, 30, 31, 32, 77, 87
    regulation of, 13
cirrhosis, 16, 60, 61, 62, 64, 66–7,
        78, 83, 90, 94
    primary biliary, 16, 77–8
coma, 24, 62
confusion, 24, 82
contraceptive pill, 37
CT scan, 83, 84, 93

delirium tremens, 65
depression, 24, 71
diabetes, 16, 25
diagnosing gallstones, 42–6
diarrhoea, 23, 26, 69, 77
diet and gallstones, 38, 51–2
disulfiram tablets (Antabuse), 61,
        65
drugs
    and alcoholism, 65, 66, 79
    and gallstones, 39, 47, 52, 54,
        55
    and liver disease, 16, 68, 70, 72,
        78, 80, 83
duodenum, 9, 10, 23
dye, injecting, 43–4, 49, 93
Ebola fever, 74
electrolytes, 88
endoscopy, 43-4, 54
enzymes, 17, 26, 32, 61–2, 78, 86

ether treatment, 56–7

fats, absorption of, 11, 17, 28–9, 77
fluid, 22, 82, 90

gallbladder, 7, 9
  functions of, 10
  inflammation of, 21, 41
  removal of, 25
  see also gallstones
gallstones, 25, 27–9
  in bile ducts, 21, 25, 27, 28, 46
  causes of, 34–41
  crushing, 55
  detection of, 42–6
  dissolving, 52–3, 54, 55
  formation of, 31–2
  people at risk, 34–7
  symptoms of, 25, 26, 27, 40–1
  treatment for, 47–57
  types of, 32–3
Gilbert's syndrome, 20, 21
glandular fever, 16, 75, 89
globulin, 70, 87
hepatitis, 16, 82
  A (infectious), 68–71, 89
  alcoholic, 62
  B, 71–3, 83, 89
  chronic active, 16, 78
  delta, 73
  non-A non-B, 74, 89
hepatoma see cancer, liver
herbs, 16, 81
hormones, 13, 14, 80

immunisation, 68, 70, 72, 74
infections, 16, 18, 28, 68–76, 88–9
insulin, 7, 17, 25
isotope scan, 43, 64, 84, 94
itch, 23, 69, 77, 78, 80

jaundice, 14, 46, 62, 76, 85, 90, 91
  causes of, 19–21, 80
  in infants, 75
  obstructive, 27, 40–1

lasers, 56
lecithin, 30, 31
liver
  abscess, 16, 76
  and alcohol, 58–67

anatomy of, 7–9
auto-immune disease, 16, 77–8
biopsy, 64, 65, 77, 84, 90, 92
causes of damage, 15–16,
  19–21
functions of, 7, 11–15
inflammation of, 21
symptoms of disease, 85–6, 91
tests for disease, 85–9
transplants, 16, 75, 78, 82, 83
treatment of failure, 82
and viruses, 68–76, 88–9

Marburg disease, 74
mental problems, 24, 66, 85

oral cholecystogram, 43, 52

pain, 25, 26, 27, 40, 41
  treatment for, 47
pancreas, 7, 10
  functions of, 17
  inflammation of, 25–6
pancreatitis, acute, 25, 27, 41
pancreatitis, chronic, 26
paracetamol, 14, 16, 79–80, 82
phospholipids, 30, 31
pigments, 11, 14, 19
pregnancy, 36
prostaglandins, 47

salt, 22, 66, 88
soundwaves, 56
spleen, 16, 22, 75, 85, 94
  functions of, 18
stools, 11, 20, 21, 23
surgery
  for gallstones, 25, 26, 48–51, 91
  liver see transplants
  pancreas, 26
symptoms
  of alcohol abuse, 62–3
  of gallstones, 25, 26, 27, 40–1
  of liver disease, 85–6, 91
  lack of, 40

tests
  blood, 44, 69, 78, 86
  for gallstones, 42–6, 49, 93
  liver function, 64, 85–9, 95
  see also biopsy

tranquillisers, 80
transplants, liver, 16, 75, 78, 82, 83
treatment
  for alcoholism, 65
  of auto-immune disease, 8
  of gallstones, 47–57, 91
  of hepatitis, 69, 72, 78
  of liver cancer, 83
  of liver failure, 82
  for pain, 47
  surgical, 25, 26, 48–51, 75, 91
  see also drugs; transplants

ulcers, 23, 66
ultrasound, 42, 43, 45, 52, 53, 84,
    92, 94
urea, 87

viruses and liver disease, 68–76,
    88–9
vitamin A, 11, 77
vitamin B, 15, 23
vitamin D, 11, 77
vitamin K, 11, 22, 66, 77

weight and gallstones, 37
Weil's disease, 76
women and gallstones, 36–7

X rays, 43, 44, 45, 93, 94

yellow colouring, 19, 21, 40, 91–2
yellow fever, 16, 74